Herbal
Remedies

Survival Guide

Empower Your Health with Plants and
Herbs—From Daily Wellness to
Crisis Recovery

By

ENDURE ELITE

The information in this book is not intended to replace medical advice. Please consult your doctor before starting any herbal medicine regime, especially if you are pregnant, breastfeeding, have a medical condition, are taking any medication, or plan to have blood tests or surgery.

Endure Elite offers a variety of books that teach you the essential skills to thrive—no matter what life throws your way—from your health and wellness priorities to survival skills. We're experts at providing education, resources, and practical advice that suits everyone, whether you're just starting out or you're a self-sufficient, seasoned pro. Our approach is pragmatic and user-friendly, featuring reliable, scientifically validated health and wellness strategies and credible survival methods that will provide you with the skills, confidence, and resilience to prepare for and master any situation or environment.

TABLE OF CONTENTS

38 page herbal profile and usage guide!

Instant Access to Over 70 Herbal Profiles in an Online & Printable PDF Format (A $25 Value)

Or go to tinyurl.com/**EndureHerb**

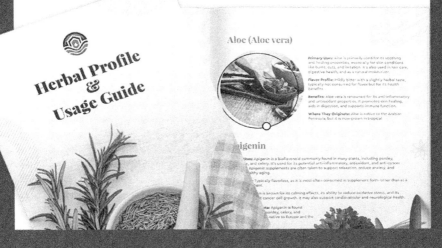

"In the midst of death, life persists. In the midst of untruth, truth persists. In the midst of darkness, light persists."

— MAHATMA GANDHI

INTRODUCTION

When you think about our distant ancestors, what do you picture? A bunch of knuckle-dragging cavemen with spears, hunting wild game, and sitting around a fire, gnawing bones? Our stone-age predecessors were hunter-gatherers, and we now have archaeological evidence that they used powerful botanical ingredients for food, clothing, and medicine. At seven different archaeological sites in the Middle East, dating back to the Middle and Later Paleolithic era (a time frame spanning 800,000 years to ten thousand years ago), archaeologists identified 212 plant species, of which 60 percent were a mix of edible and medicinal, and 15 percent were non-edible (bitter, with low nutritional value), but known to have medicinal power.

The same archaeologists made another intriguing find in Spain when they discovered a fifty-thousand-year-old Neanderthal woman with a tooth abscess. Analysis of her dental plaque revealed yarrow, chamomile, and poplar—all plants that possess potent herbal ingredients confirmed by modern scientists. For example, poplar contains salicylic acid, the active pain-killing ingredient in aspirin, and a natural penicillin-like antibiotic (Alex 2019).

After I experienced a debilitating health crisis and started learning about traditional herbal medicine, I pictured that chart of evolution from apes to Homo sapiens, and I thought about the wisdom we've lost in that evolutionary march through time. Don't get me wrong; I'm no Luddite. I like a lot of things about modern life. But when you're facing a health crisis, it's hard to find any light.

It was one of the darkest days of my life. I woke up before dawn with stabbing pain in my abdomen. I was twenty-two, and my first thought was, "I'm going to die today." I called 911, curled up in a ball, and waited for the sound of sirens. At the hospital, they did some tests and found out that my gallbladder was overworked and irreversibly scarred; it was said to be the type of damaged bladder you'd expect to find in a fifty-year-old! My gallbladder had to be removed, and soon after that, I developed a gluten allergy and excruciatingly painful digestive tract issues. My doctor suspected Crohn's disease, and I had to go through so many medical tests to figure out what was wrong with me. I discovered that I have a gluten allergy, and I realized that I would have to radically alter my diet and my lifestyle. It was so stressful, and I felt like I had no control over my body and my mind. I read about the medications for gastrointestinal illnesses and found out that they have many debilitating side effects and can even cause new digestive tract problems (Philpott 2014). I wanted natural, holistic options, and in the past, I'd dabbled with traditional medicines, but I didn't always find them effective, and I was skeptical about all the so-called miracle cures. I knew that I had to do something proactive. I had to find some light.

I decided to devote myself to learning about herbalism. I did tons of research and took a journey of discovery, starting with ancient treatments and analyzing the latest medical research about botanicals. Along the way, I found out that about 60 percent of the world's population still relies on herbal medicine, and 80 percent of people in developing countries use plant-based treatments almost exclusively for their essential health care needs (Robinson 2011).

In the Western world, we've lost so much of that ancient wisdom. Today, only 25 percent of medical drugs come from natural sources. While there are an estimated 300,000 plant species, only about 15 percent of them have been evaluated as potential pharmaceuticals (Palhares 2015).

We tend to rely heavily on pharmaceutical drugs, which may be vital for many health issues but can often cause serious or deadly side effects. In the US, more than two million people have serious adverse reactions to medications, and 100,000 people die from medications, making it one of the leading causes of illness and mortality (Eldridge 2023). Medications can interact with other drugs, foods, vitamins, minerals, and herbal ingredients so that medications are either less effective or have too much potency.

With the rising popularity of plant-based medicines, scientific research has focused increasingly on applying modern medical protocols to herbal medicine research by identifying, purifying, and standardizing the chemical constituents and conducting clinical trials with people to test for efficacy and safety (Firenzuoli 2007). This is complex research because the chemical composition of plants varies due to several factors: the botanical species and the specific geographic region where that species is grown; the part of the plant used (such as seed, flower, leaf, or root); the date of harvest; and the way the plant is preserved and stored.

I'll show you how to draw on ancient wisdom and modern medical research so that you can customize your health and wellness needs, make your own sustainable, eco-friendly food recipes and herbal remedies, and become less reliant on Big Food and Big Pharma—two industries implicated in global pollution and the ongoing climate change crisis. That's why I started on this journey. I became a herbalist to improve my health, rely less on medical drugs and supermarket foods, and take back control of my life. Along the way, I realized that herbal medicine is also good for the planet.

The pharmaceutical industry's ecological footprint is huge. Factories use a lot of water and as much as triple the energy consumption as the average office space. About 15 percent of modern health care products generate hazardous waste during the production process, which contaminates water, land and the air we breathe with an estimated 300 million tons of plastic, radioactive waste and many chemicals, including concentrated "active pharmaceutical ingredients" (APIs) and volatile organic compounds (VOCs), causing pollution to communities and sewage treatment facilities near factories. Pharma also generates approximately fifty-two megatons of CO_2—equal to the greenhouse gas emissions of eleven million cars. Medical drugs are engineered to be long-lasting, so the compounds—antibiotics, chemotherapy drugs, hormones, and mood-altering drugs—are known as persistent pharmaceutical pollutants because they stick around in the environment for a long time, jeopardizing wild animals, ecosystems, and human life. For example, antibiotic-resistant bacterial infections have already led to five million deaths, and mortality is estimated to double by 2050.

The use of plants and botanicals—as both our food and our medicine—literally saves lives. But with herbal medicine, we also need to be mindful to practice sustainability to protect our planet's ecosystems. Scientists estimate that 25 percent of plant species could vanish within the next three decades, and one in five popular medicinal plants will go extinct due to overharvesting. In China, where 70 percent of medicine is derived from plants, half of these plants have disappeared in the past two decades (Thomas 2021).

In this book, I'll provide you with the essential information about cultivating a thriving, sustainable home herbal garden that feeds your body, mind and spirit so that you have a practical, user-friendly, holistic approach to herbalism. I'll show you how to grow, harvest and preserve plants and create your own herbal remedies for yourself and all your loved ones, from children to seniors. I'll supply safe, effective and economical options that can help supercharge your health and prevent and treat a diversity of health issues—everything from insect bites to allergies to anxiety, depression and the top chronic conditions and diseases, including cancers and cardiovascular disorders. We'll cut through the hype, dubious claims, and complex medical information so that you have the knowledge, skills, and confidence to become a self-sufficient herbalist with an incredible garden of wellness at your fingertips.

The Eight Steps to Self-Empowerment

This book will unlock the secrets to optimal health and self-empowerment by blending the ancient wisdom of herbal and plant-based medicine with validation from modern science and up-to-date resources, research, and tips from experts. My method features a dynamic, practical, and actionable eight-step holistic plan that will help you grow and produce your own remedies, master herbal medicine, become self-sufficient and thrive—whatever happens in the future. Each chapter includes advice and research from our ancient ancestors, traditional healers, herbal medicine experts, and the latest medical science, along with the key techniques for growing, harvesting, storing and utilizing plant and herb-based remedies. I'll provide you with many step-by-step guides and recipes to make your own safe and effective herbal remedies so that your pantry, medicine cabinet, and entire home are stocked with homemade products that are sustainable, eco-friendly, and healthy—for you and the planet.

H: History of Herbs: From ancient times to the present day, this chapter will cover the significant developments and setbacks in herbal medicine, the birth of the pharmaceutical industry, and the most up-to-date medical science, which has confirmed and validated the potency, efficacy, and safety of so many ancient herbal medicines. We'll reconnect with the ancient, time-honored wisdom of our ancestors, whose knowledge still endures in many modern cultures but has unfortunately been lost to much of the Western world, dominated by unsustainable industries that can negatively impact our health and harm our planet, including Big Pharma and Big Food. We'll rediscover the power and sustainability of these remedies, learn about the seven key plant phytonutrients, and dig into why—and how—herbal medicines can supercharge your health and wellness. We'll help you customize your remedies to your needs, those of your family and loved ones, and our imperiled ecosystem.

O: Optimize Your Health and Wellness: This chapter will cover the key eco-friendly plants and superfoods that are good for you and the planet, in contrast to the Big Pharma and Big Food industries, both of which have massive ecological footprints and many health implications. I'll introduce you to some of the best herbal medicines for preventing and treating many diseases, health disorders, and chronic conditions based on both ancient wisdom and modern scientific evidence. We'll also cover the ideal plants for cleansing, detoxing, and boosting energy, cognition, and the immune system.

L: Learn About the Essential Plants and Herbs For Your First Aid Kit: To help you become self-sufficient and master your survival skills, I'll discuss the key powerful herbal remedies for your medicine cabinet, including plants that help treat headaches, toothaches, joint pain, cuts, burns, stings, and allergies.

I: Invigorate Your Health: This chapter will discuss the ideal phytonutrient-loaded plants and herbs to help prevent and treat the most common diseases and chronic conditions linked to mortality, including cardiovascular diseases, cancer, respiratory disorders, autoimmune conditions, cognitive age-related diseases, including Alzheimer's and dementia, along with herbal options that support medical therapies and may reduce treatment-related side effects to help you heal.

S: Step-by-Step Guide to Creating Your Own Organic, Eco-friendly Garden: This chapter will teach you to make safe, effective herbal remedies, starting from scratch with a seedling garden of your preferred plant and herb seeds, transplanting tips, and harvesting and storage techniques.

T: Take Control of Your Mental Health: This chapter will look at potent treatments and herbal medicines backed by modern clinical research to enhance your mood and provide peace of mind and emotional balance. These natural remedies, in contrast to some pharmaceutical drugs that often cause adverse effects, may reduce anxiety, stress, depression, and emotional trauma. We'll also dive into the fascinating brain-gut connection that's only recently been found to link mental health with the digestive system's microbiome, and I'll provide the ideal prebiotic, probiotic and postbiotic plants and foods to cultivate a healthy gut. We'll also feed the soul, learning about the ancient spiritual and ritual practices that relied on plant and herbal remedies to forge a healthy mind-body-spirit connection and realign us with the natural world.

I: Ignite Your Creativity: This chapter will teach you to incorporate herbs and plants into all aspects of your life with step-by-step guides to making organic herbal remedies, including infusions, decoctions, tinctures and essential oils, and organic, DIY personal care and household cleaning options—soaps, laundry detergents, and shampoo— that are economical, chemical-free, and beneficial to us and the planet, in contrast to the conventional products and even products labeled "organic," which are known to cause health problems and environmental damage.

C: Cultivate and Grow Your Herbal Garden Skills: This chapter will teach you to enhance your garden and enrich your community's biodiversity with ideal native and pollinator-friendly plants. We will also offer tips for growing deeper roots in your community. We'll also look at safe, eco-friendly foraging and wildcrafting for plants and herbs, tips on shopping for budget-friendly organic foods, and resources to help you grow your herbal medicine network, including neighborhood and community greening ideas, co-operative farmer's markets, supporting local, eco-friendly agricultural farms and herbalists, connecting with herbal and plant-based enthusiasts and experts around the world, and keeping up-to-date on regional and global traditional medicine initiatives.

Lighting the Path to Sustainable, Eco-friendly Health and Wellness

Herbal medicine provided the light I needed to find my path out of the darkness of a health crisis and not just survive it—but thrive. But that's just the start of the journey. I'm still learning, and in the spirit of our wise ancestors, the more I know, the more I'm humbled and curious to learn more. And the more I learn, the stronger my connections become—to my loved ones, to my community, and to the natural world. By following my HOLISTIC step-by-step method, you too can have the keys to unlock the door to a self-empowered, self-sufficient, future-proof life of great health and well-being—for you and the ecosystem!

Before we get started, please remember that herbal remedies, either alone or in combination with other plants and foods or pharmaceutical interventions (including drugs that require blood test monitoring or surgical anesthesia), can cause allergies, serious adverse effects, and blood test results that can increase or decrease the potency, efficacy and side effects of drug therapies (O'Leary 2011). It's imperative that you talk to a doctor before starting a herbal regimen, particularly if you're taking medications, have any pre-existing health conditions, are pregnant or breastfeeding (or plan on becoming pregnant in the near future), planning to have surgery in the near future, or if you're providing herbal medicines to children.

"The natural healing force within each one of us is the greatest force in getting well. Our food should be our medicine, and our medicine should be our food."

– HIPPOCRATES

CHAPTER ONE

The History of Herbal Medicine

The Past, Present and Future of Plant-Based Medicine

L et's tap into the ancient and constantly evolving wisdom of our ancestors and go back in time to the fifty-thousand-year-old Neanderthal to kick off this chapter about the fascinating history of herbal medicine. But instead of picturing a chart of our continual evolution into intelligent humans with great posture, think about it like a roller coaster ride with a lot of ups and downs, hairpin turns, and the occasional terrified screams of tortured witches and naturopathic practitioners.

Sadly, in the Western world, we've lost much of our ancient collective wisdom, and our industrial and pharmaceutical industries have spread across the globe like a toxic invader species, jeopardizing the planet and creating a global health care crisis. But there's a silver lining to this story. I don't want to give a spoiler, so I'll just say that by the end of this chapter, you'll learn the science of the secret life of plants and discover why and how they're such powerful medicines. It turns out, we are a lot like what we eat!

As the old saying goes, if we don't learn from history, we're doomed to repeat the mistakes of the past. However, we can doom-proof our future by leaning on the wisdom and enthusiasm for plant-based medicines, avoiding the follies of the recent past and the predicted future cataclysms.

Anthropologists believe our ancient predecessors used trial and error to learn which plants could provide sustenance, soothe common ailments, and treat diseases, and they passed that wisdom on to the next generation. They probably also observed the customs of animals, including our closest relatives, chimpanzees. Recent research confirmed that chimps eat many herbal remedies, including antibacterial, anti-inflammatory plants, to treat tapeworms, gastrointestinal issues, and pain and injury-related swelling (Kuta 2024).

Going on the Record

It's hard to pinpoint the date that our distant relatives became adept at herbal medicine because there was no written record until it was etched in clay tablets over five thousand years ago in Mesopotamia. The Sumerians recorded the first herbal recipes of more than 250 plants, including poppy, mandrake, and henbane. I highly doubt that such deep knowledge appeared out of nowhere. In China circa 2,500 BCE, Emperor Shen Nung wrote a book featuring 365 medicinal plants still used today, such as ginseng, cinnamon bark, and ephedra (Petrovsca 2012). By 1500 BCE, the ancient Egyptians had a list of 850 herbal medicines used to treat a diversity of specialties, including gynecology, mental health, and dentistry, featuring many herbal recipes that we still rely on today, including garlic, cumin, coriander, and aloe. Africa, India, and Babylon also had ancient wisdom about herbs, which is still prized today. In India, Ayurvedic texts date back to 400 BCE, noting hundreds of herbal remedies still used today, such as ashwagandha and turmeric (Herbal Academy, n.d.).

At about the same time, in Greece, a doctor named Hippocrates documented 300 medicines and linked them to specific illnesses, including garlic for intestinal parasites and as a diuretic (Petrovska 2012). Hippocrates believed that illness is the result of physical issues in the body, which broke from the conventional theory that illness was due to the wrath of the gods

(Timmons 2023). It would take centuries for the separation of church and medicine to become popular in the Western world. In the meantime, herbalists were often accused of witchcraft, and when the Romans conquered Greece, they banned all the medical books about herbalism. But throughout the medieval era, Europeans created translations and handwritten copies of ancient texts and practices, which helped spread knowledge. The invention of the printing press put this ancient and evolving wisdom in the hands of citizens around the world, including the first English language book about botanical medicine, the *Grete Herball*, which was published in the 1500s.

Unfortunately, the rising popularity of herbal medicine in the Western world riled many physicians who wanted to maintain strict control of this powerful information. In the mid-1600s, a London-based herbalist named Nicholas Culpeper, who studied at Cambridge to become a doctor but chose to become an apothecary instead, published a book about botanical medicines and provided citizens with free books and free treatments. For that, he was persecuted, imprisoned, and tried for witchcraft. Luckily, his book made it to North America, where colonists also learned about ancient Indigenous practices and knowledge from African slaves. Yet, herbalists continued to lock horns with physicians who preferred invasive methods like bloodletting and using toxic minerals like mercury and arsenic (Herbal Academy n.d.).

Across the pond, pre-conquest Indigenous Americans and ancient Mesoamerican civilizations in Mexico and Central and South America had deep knowledge of botanical medicine and a holistic approach to health and wellness. Indigenous Navajo healers didn't just treat the body; they saw each person as a mind and a spirit, interconnected with the community, other animals and plants, the planet, and the entire universe. For many Indigenous American cultures, good medicine involves herbal medicines and many other traditional healing methods, including fasting, rituals, meditation, sweat lodge ceremonies, and maintaining harmony with the natural world (Redvers 2020). Sadly, their conquistadors didn't share their reverence for nature and nurture.

The Birth of Big Pharma

Manufactured drugs first appeared in the 19th century and relied primarily on plant ingredients. For example, one of the first drugs on the market was aspirin, derived from salicin, isolated from salix alba (Veeresham 2012). At the same time, powerful medical associations were established, including the American Medical Association, which standardized medical education, and by 1935, the majority of medical schools that practiced naturopathic medicine were consolidated with AMA-friendly universities or shut down (McFarling 2021.) In the UK, the *Pharmacies and Medicines Act* prevented herbalists from supplying patients with botanicals (Herbal Academy n.d.). It wasn't until the 1960s that herbal medicine became popular once again in Western countries and was eventually re-integrated with conventional medicine and modern pharmaceuticals, which still relied on plants for 50 percent of all approved drugs. Researchers have also noted that 80 percent of modern plant-derived drugs are used to treat the same conditions as the ancient herbal treatments (Veeresham 2012).

Pharmaceutical offshoots of plants, which are powerful, vital, and affordable compounds, have since been used to treat many cancers, cardiovascular and liver diseases, Parkinson's disease, Alzheimer's, and, ironically, drug-resistant infections. In 2000, the WHO listed more than 250 essential drugs, of which 11 percent originated from flowering plants (Veeresham 2012). Yet today, while it's estimated that there are more than 250,000 species of plants, including more than 600 anticancer plant compounds (50 percent of all anticancer agents), only 10 percent of these species have been investigated for pharmaceutical products (Muhammad 2022).

In the past decade, the WHO has made it a priority to integrate traditional and complementary medicine (T&CM) with national health care systems, noting that "health systems around the world are experiencing increased illness and escalating health care costs." At the same time, our use of pharmaceutical drugs has steadily increased by 14 percent between 2018 and 2023—that's an increase of 414 billion daily doses, and it's projected to double by 2028 (IQVIA 2024). Yet only one-tenth of new drugs approved by the FDA are proven to be more effective, and only one-third are studied post-approval, which is concerning because these post-approval studies are the most reliable way to gauge efficacy and safety in the real world. For example, recent research found that thirty-one of thirty-six approved cancer drugs didn't have a positive impact on survival (Pease 2017).

The WHO highlighted that these costs could be offset by traditional medicine (TM), improving treatment efficacy, health and longevity, and individualizing care while reducing the economic burden. This 2013 WHO strategy acknowledged increased global investment in TM education, accreditation, and research and development and highlighted the WHO's commitment to "support Member States in developing proactive policies and implementing action plans that will strengthen the role TM plays in keeping populations healthy."

Speaking at a 2013 conference on TM, WHO Director-General Dr. Margaret Chan stated that "traditional medicines, of proven quality, safety, and efficacy, contribute to the goal of ensuring that all people have access to care. For many millions of people, herbal medicines, traditional treatments, and traditional practitioners are the main source of health care and sometimes the only source of care. This is care that is close to homes, accessible, and affordable. It is also culturally acceptable and trusted by large numbers of people. The affordability of most traditional medicines makes them all the more attractive at a time of soaring health care costs and nearly universal austerity. Traditional medicine also stands out as a way of coping with the relentless rise of chronic non-communicable diseases" (World Health Organization 2013).

I hope you take this statement as a rallying call to embrace traditional herbal remedies and curtail our reliance on Big Pharma. As I said, this history lesson isn't all doom and gloom. Science has helped unlock the secret life of plants and herbs and validated the potency of so many plants and herbs. In future chapters, we'll dig into more details about herbal options, but let's start by learning about the seven key phytonutrients linked to optimal health and wellness.

You Are What You Eat

In many ways, plants are just like us. They have an immune system and produce phytonutrients with powerful antioxidants, protecting them from parasites, bacteria, fungi, viruses, and damage caused by environmental toxins. Antioxidants also neutralize free radicals linked to many diseases and disorders, including cancer and heart disease. Antioxidants keep free radicals in check so that they don't cause oxidative stress, which can damage and destroy our cells and our DNA. Phytonutrients are found in all our plant-based foods and drinks—fruits, veggies, beans, grains, nuts, herbs, spices, tea, and coffee—and they give plants and foods their signature colors, flavors, and aromas. They also help plants produce pollen, protection from insects and pests, and ultraviolet light (Monjotin 2022).

Validating Traditional Medicine with Modern Medical Research

Studies have consistently found that high intake of plant-based foods and herbal medicines are linked to a longer life and lower risks of diseases. They help balance the immune system so that it doesn't tip the scales towards low reactions (which can increase the risk of viral and bacterial infections) or high reactions, which can lead to chronic inflammation and inflammatory diseases. They also help prevent and treat cardiovascular diseases and many cancers by protecting DNA from damage, repairing genes, helping eradicate abnormal cells in the body and the brain, and producing antioxidants (UCLA Health 2023).

In modern medical research, botanical ingredients like pharmaceutical drugs derived from plants are tested for efficacy and safety, starting with the isolation of a specific plant part to identify its active chemical ingredients, predict how we'll absorb, distribute, metabolize, and excrete that substance, and determine whether it's toxic (Gu 2024). The next step is calculating safety and efficacy, first with preclinical research (lab and animal testing) and then with three phases of clinical trials with people, ideally comparing the treatment group to a control group that receives no treatment or a placebo. Researchers start with small groups to calculate safety and dosage and then scale up to three thousand people, monitoring side effects and weighing the benefits against the risks. The FDA approves only one in four compounds or drugs, and if approved, the drug goes through more clinical trials with more than three thousand people to provide extra safety monitoring (FDA 2018). But as I mentioned earlier, once a medication is approved, only one-third are actually studied among large, diverse populations. That's why it's always wise to start with a low dose of herbal medicine, look out for side effects, and then increase gradually to higher therapeutic doses.

Phytonutrients

Modern scientists have identified thousands of phytochemicals in plants and plant-based foods, and more than twenty-five thousand papers have been published in scientific journals about their specific health benefits. But with all clinical research (including conventional medicine and pharmaceutical clinical trials) not all studies are equally rigorous, high-quality, evidence-based and unbiased. To identify the best research, scientists conduct systematic reviews by assessing every published study on a specific topic, analyzing the quality of the data, and eliminating studies that deviate from standard protocols in clinical research and lack valid, reliable, objective information. The benefit of a systematic review is that it looks at thousands of studies published in peer-reviewed medical journals conducted by researchers all over the world and provides a comprehensive summary of the most reliable research results (Ahn 2018).

There are thousands of systematic reviews about the health benefits of plant-based phytonutrients. Let's take a look at one from 2022 by French researchers that reviewed studies published about the health benefits of key phytonutrients linked to disease prevention and reduced mortality— as anti-inflammatory, antimicrobial, anticancer and antioxidants. They identified more than twenty-three thousand articles, filtered out the significant majority, and ultimately analyzed only seventy-four articles that met the criteria of robust, reliable research. The researchers did a deep dive into these studies, crunched all the numbers, and provided a list of seven key phytonutrients that benefit health and longevity (Monjotin 2022). Below is a highlight of their key findings, including dietary sources.

Phenolic Acids

These nutrients reduce osteoarthritis-related pain and improve cognitive function, including memory. Dietary sources of phenolic acids include cereals and wheat flour, artichokes, onions, kiwis, berries, apples, citrus fruits, and caffeine. Phenolic acids are also produced by metabolizing other polyphenols.

Flavonoids

Flavonoids strengthen the immune system, protect against colds and flu, reduce insomnia and stress, improve cognitive function and digestive health, reduce constipation and nausea in chemotherapy patients, improve liver function, reduce symptoms of rheumatoid arthritis, and prevent menopausal osteoporosis by increasing bone density. These phytonutrients also belong to the polyphenol family. The main dietary sources include many plants colored red, yellow, and purple, including apples, citrus fruits, tomatoes, pears, olives, cabbage, lettuce, celery, onions, tea, and red wine.

Anthocyanins

With their strong anti-inflammatory effects, anthocyanins help manage ulcerative colitis, reduce tumor necrosis in lymph nodes and improve sleep, energy levels, and both physical and cognitive performance (including improved memory and reduced anxiety and depression in elderly people). These are most commonly found in red, pink, blue, orange, and purple-colored fruits and veggies, such as cherries, berries, plums, eggplant, red cabbage, and red wine, and root veggies like beets, radishes, red onion bulbs.

Tannins

Another immune system powerhouse, tannins boost energy, help curb flu symptoms and allergies, and ease digestive issues, including constipation and irritable bowel syndrome-related pain and discomfort. High tannin sources include tea, wine, plums, barley seeds, cocoa beans, carob beans, and pomegranate bark.

Organosulfur Compounds

A strong antiviral immune system booster linked to improved liver function, these compounds are also known to reduce joint pain and stiffness and make an ideal antioxidant for the digestive tract. They're found in cruciferous veggies like broccoli, cabbage, turnips, black radish, mustard, and garlic.

Carotenoids

Another anti-inflammatory super-phyto, they're an ideal preventative against chronic joint disorders and are linked to improved muscle strength and power. They can also reduce cortisol levels and mood-related issues, including anxiety, improve cognitive function (especially concentration, alertness and memory), and relieve headaches. Carotenoids are found in many plants, particularly yellow, orange, and red dietary sources and leafy greens. High sources of carotenoids include citrus fruits, carrots, peppers, spinach, tomatoes, parsley, basil, saffron, lettuce, arugula, broccoli, kale, brussels sprouts, squash, sweet potato, seeds, and mushrooms.

Caffeine

Despite the concern that caffeine can increase stress levels, research has found that daily caffeine consumption (a max of 400 ml/day) can actually decrease stress and curb depression, as well as improving respiratory function in people with asthma. You'll find it in coffee, tea, kola nuts, and guarana seeds.

Phytonutrient Panacea

A plant or herb may contain many of the above phytochemicals and dozens, if not hundreds, of other chemical compounds. For example, moringa, known as the drumstick tree and the horseradish tree, contains 110 bioactive chemicals. These chemicals are known to be anti-inflammatory, antioxidant, antihypertensive, anticancer, antimicrobial, antidiabetic, analgesic, prebiotic and immunomodulatory. Moringa is also a great source of iron, containing seventeen fatty acids and all the essential amino acids. Added perks include that it's inexpensive to cultivate and thrives year-round, including in the dry season (Camilleri 2024).

As I mentioned earlier, in upcoming chapters, I'll highlight many more potent herbs and plants linked to optimal health. I also highly recommend that you get your hands on some of the books written by past herbal medicine practitioners, like Dr. Culpeper. To look at medical research, check out the latest published medical research about specific herbal plants that have been found effective in preventing and treating your specific health conditions. A great place to start is the NIH National Library of Medicine. You can type the name of any herbal compound into the search engine to find peer-reviewed research published in thousands of journals around the world at https://pubmed.ncbi.nlm.nih.gov/.

NIH also has a mobile app called HerbList, where you can search popular herbal remedies, scientific studies, and research-based information on safety, efficacy and side effects. You can access it via Apple or Google Play (NIH 2018).

Safety First

The majority of healthy people can enjoy the above-cited whole food sources as part of a well-balanced diet without worrying about adverse effects, but speak to your doctor first if you're taking medications that interact with specific foods, you have a medical condition, allergies to specific foods or chemicals, or you're pregnant or breastfeeding.

I hope that after reading about the good, bad and sometimes ugly evolution of herbal medicine, you're motivated to start relying less on conventional medicine and more on plant-based and herbal remedies that have stood the test of time *and* science. Luckily, we can still draw from the wisdom of traditional and herbal medicine pioneers, some of whom risked *their* lives to keep that wisdom alive and available to the public. Without their knowledge, I might still e lost in the labyrinth of a health care crisis. I hope that by learning about the potent nutrients and chemicals in plants and herbs, you draw the same inspiration and are keen to get your hands dirty and grow your own garden of medicinal plants.

In the next chapter, we'll turn the spotlight on the many environmentally unsustainable practices in the food industry and explore the alternative path of eco-friendly, optimal plant-based medicines for preventing and treating common diseases and chronic conditions. We'll also dig into the ideal herbal remedies for cleansing, detoxing, and boosting energy, cognition, and immune systems.

"The health of a nation is directly tied to the health of its food system."

— WENDELL BARRY

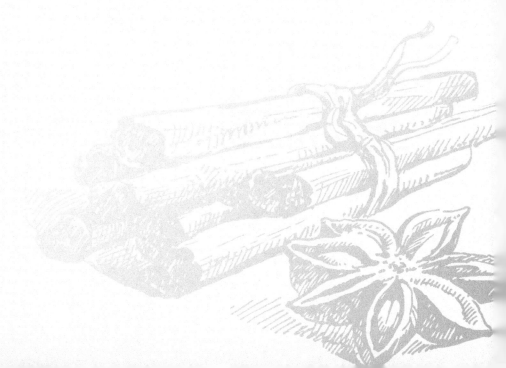

CHAPTER TWO

Optimize Your Health

Eco-friendly Herbal Medicines

Today's supermarket is a bizarre place. It has morphed from a locally owned grocery store to a gigantic fluorescent box where you can get tires, furniture and appliances, and many brightly packaged food-like products, but not much actual food. It's easy to get lost and disillusioned in there.

This chapter will help you find a way out of the Big Food maze and provide a path to a better life with real food that's organic and sustainable—a win-win for you and the planet! By contrast, the ecological footprint of the traditional food industry is massive. Food production accounts for 26 percent of global emissions. From source to landfill, each stage of the process is environmentally harmful to the planet. The rising global population has led to unsustainable mass agriculture methods, including 80 percent of deforestation, 70 percent of the pollution of freshwater sources, and the use of harmful pesticides and herbicides that deplete the nutritional properties of food and soil nutrients (Davison 2024).

These foods are typically wrapped in single-use packaging, which accounts for about one-third of all global packaging, generating a total of 12.5 million tons of plastic waste (FAO 2023.) This food waste ends up in landfills and accounts for 58 percent of landfill gas that pollutes the earth, oceans, and air (EPA 2023). Much of the packaging for our food products, from plastic bottles to plastic sheets to polystyrene, isn't biodegradable or recyclable and causes long-term degradation of the planet and the oceans, jeopardizing land and marine species. According to the UN, agriculture has led to the risk of extinction for 86 percent of animal species (UNEP 2021).

In the US, Big Food generates 10 percent of total global emissions (EPA 2022). Our increasing demand for every food year-round has led to a spike in global exports from many far-flung countries so that we can eat their fruits and veggies on demand. That transport released twice as much greenhouse gases as Big Food production (Davison 2024).

From source to grocery store, Big Food requires a lot of energy. The next time you go to the supermarket and stroll past the giant fridges and freezers packed with fruits and vegetables, think about the fact that your local supermarket emits the carbon of three hundred cars per year (Chung 2023). In the US, when wasted food hits the landfill and rots, it generates fifty-five million metric tons of CO_2 and 61 percent of methane gas emissions (EPA 2023).

All of that pollution is harmful to us, too. We drink these microplastics—one-quarter of a million are in a single liter of bottled water—and our water sources are contaminated by pesticides and herbicides linked to many deadly diseases, including cancer (Davison 2024).

About half of the world's soil is degraded from pollution and overharvesting (Perry 2018), and there are human rights costs, too, including exploitative and unsafe labor practices with agricultural workers and the conversion of biodiverse regions and countries that traditionally relied on medicinal plants (Morrison 2023). Fortunately, today, eco-conscious consumers and local growers are forging a demand for organic, environmentally friendly and sustainable food products that are transforming the way we think about and produce our food (WEF 2021). There's also been a growing demand for herbal supplements, and many stores are bursting with options, but quantity doesn't typically equate with quality.

Low Quality and Toxic Herbal Supplements

Today, the herbal supplement industry is booming, but even these plants aren't immune to adulteration during agricultural production and processing. Industry testing has found chemicals, heavy metals, pesticides, toxic microbes, prescription medications and over-the-counter (OTC) drugs, other plants, and additives in herbal supplements. Many of these contaminants are born from pollution, poor soil quality, chemicals in fertilizers, and water contamination; others are added during the manufacturing process as fillers and to increase the potency of so-called plant-based supplements. For example, the California Department of Health Services Food and Drug Branch did a study on more than two hundred plant-based patented medicines from retail herbal stores and found that 7 percent contained undeclared pharmaceuticals, including ephedrine, chlorpheniramine, methyltestosterone, and phenacetin, all of which cause increased energy. They also found that 14 percent contained mercury and arsenic (Hassen 2022).

Another report by US researchers stated that "financially motivated adulteration of spices is a long-standing and important public health problem worldwide." They found that state spot checks of imported products, particularly turmeric and curry powder, sold by US companies and farmer's markets had high concentrations of lead chromate, leading to recalls. Yet the FDA has no guidelines for maximum lead levels in spices, so the scientists had to use the allowable level in candy, finding that half of their samples of turmeric exceeded that level. The researchers concluded the lead wasn't just coming from the soil during growth, citing reports that farmers use lead to brighten the color of turmeric (Cowell 2017).

There are many reasons that herbal products are ineffective and even toxic, including (Bloom Institute 2019):

▶ They are "cut and sifted," meaning they contain all the plant parts instead of the parts that contain the most potent therapeutic compounds. Take the stinging nettle, for example. The roots and leaves have good anti-inflammatory capabilities, but only the roots contain the most potent compounds.

▶ They're grown in a place that uses herbicides, pesticides, and many other sources of pollution in the local air, land, and water.

▶ The potent plant parts aren't harvested at their peak. The ideal time to harvest plant parts differs depending on the plant part and the weather conditions required for that plant part to be ready for harvest. Many plants are harvested when the leaves and stems are ready, but the flowers, seeds and roots still need time to mature.

▶ They're adulterated with other herbs, fillers, pharmaceuticals, and contaminants at processing and production facilities, or if they're sourced from other countries, they may be irradiated and fumigated for international transport.

▶ They're improperly stored and preserved, and their ideal shelf life has expired, making them less efficacious and even unsafe for consumption.

That's why I prefer to grow my own plant-based medicines. I know they're organic, high quality and sustainable because I made them myself. I'll show you how to do it, too. Let's start by returning to the traditional healers for inspiration, and then we'll get into the ideal herbal remedies for our health and well-being—and the planet's.

Plant Signatures

Many ancient cultures identified beneficial herbal remedies by their signature colors, shapes, textures, scents, and tastes. For example, Indigenous Americans linked red flowering plants with treatments for blood diseases and yellow ones to liver diseases. They also used American ginseng because it looked like a body, and many ancient cultures across the globe also used ginseng; the ancient Greeks called it *pan akos*, which means "remedy for all." In both Ayurveda and Traditional Chinese Medicine, Asian ginseng is still used as a tonic and stimulant, and modern science has since validated some of these ancient signature treatments (Durant 2014). I like to think about the signature method as a way to ground us to the earth, use all our sensory abilities to appreciate our essential interconnectedness and harness the many health benefits of plants.

Let's look at the ideal plants for preventing and treating many diseases, disorders, and chronic conditions, detoxifying and cleansing, providing energy, supporting the immune system, and boosting our cognitive and mental well-being.

I'll start with the top plants scientifically linked to treating and preventing specific health conditions. All of these plants have a long history of use in ancient cultures around the globe, and they've also been validated by conventional medical research, including the benefits and potential risks (Deering 2019).

Before we get started, please remember that plant medicines can cause allergies, interact with pharmaceutical medications, and lead to severe, even deadly, side effects. Serious complications are more likely to happen with excessive use of supplements or plant parts, so it's best to start by eating moderate amounts in your food (though some of these plants aren't tasty), and if you choose to eat or drink herbal medicine, start with a very small amount, and increase every week. And as I said before, get your doctor's approval in advance if you take any medications, have a health condition, are pregnant, breastfeeding, plan to have surgery, or want to provide herbal medicines to your children and elderly loved ones.

Turmeric

Turmeric is a pillar in Indian Ayurveda medicine. This brightly colored spice contains an important medicinal compound called curcumin. Turmeric and curcumin provide great antioxidant and anti-inflammatory support that may reduce arthritis-related pain, treat a range of skin conditions, liver disorders, and heart disease, and even prevent the growth and spread of cancer. Turmeric has low bioavailability when ingested, but piperine (a compound in black pepper) helps improve absorbency by 2000 percent (Gunnars 2023). Turmeric can cause stomach aches and is not recommended during pregnancy or nursing or for people with gallbladder or kidney problems, bleeding disorders, diabetes, or iron deficiency (Gunnars 2023; Deering 2019).

Ginger

Another ancient favorite, ginger is one of the most researched medicinal plants in medical science. We now know that the rhizome contains four hundred compounds (Pázmándi et al. 2024) that may fight diabetes, chronic pain, cognitive decline, and bad cholesterol, increase good cholesterol, and prevent various cancers, including gastrointestinal and colorectal cancer, and chemotherapy-induced side effects. It's also antimicrobial and may help fight colds and flu, aid digestion, and reduce nausea from digestive issues and menstrual pain. It's generally considered safe for moderate use but can cause heartburn, diarrhea, and mouth and throat irritation in large doses (Leech 2023).

Peppermint

This flavorful plant has been used for thousands of years in Europe and Asia, and it's packed with essential oils and nutrients. Modern research has shown that it may relieve digestive issues like IBS and reduce bloating, gas, indigestion, insomnia, seasonal allergies, migraines, menstrual cramps, insomnia, and breastfeeding pain. It's generally considered safe but can cause serious allergic reactions (Groves 2023).

Reishi Mushrooms

This fungus has a long history in TCM and among many Asian cultures. Known as "the mushroom of immortality," it has been shown to have anti-inflammatory, immunomodulatory, and chemo-preventative effects, along with the potential to suppress the development of some cancers, including colorectal and lung cancers. It's also a great energy and immune system booster. Side effects may include nausea, insomnia, and liver injury (MSKCC 2023).

Lavender

The essential oil in this fragrant, purple-flowered plant has anti-inflammatory and sedative benefits that can decrease anxiety, improve sleep, increase cognitive function, and treat migraines. Undiluted, it may negatively impact hormones and irritate skin, so if you make your own essential oil, be sure to dilute it with a carrier.

Ginkgo

Ginkgo is an essential plant in Chinese medicine. The leaves are used to make tea, capsules, tablets, and extracts. It's been shown to reduce inflammation in many diseases, including diabetes, IBS, asthma, COPD, cancer, heart disease, and stroke. It also improves brain function and eye health and treats anxiety, depression, headaches, mild-to-moderate dementia, and Alzheimer's disease. It also has many potential side effects and risks. First, ginkgo seeds are poisonous, so please don't ingest the seeds. Animal studies have also found potential links to thyroid and liver cancers, so liver enzymes should be monitored, particularly if you have a liver condition. Side effects include allergic reactions, headaches, dizziness, and stomach aches (Hill 2022; Deering 2019).

Evening Primrose Oil

This plant has bright yellow flowers, and the oil has anti-inflammatory properties that may alter hormones to treat PMS, menopause, and polycystic ovary syndrome; it's also used for many skin conditions, including atopic dermatitis and diabetic neuropathy, and it's linked to improved quality of life for people with multiple sclerosis. Be aware that it can interact with many pharmaceuticals, including blood clotting drugs, HIV meds, and lithium (Deering 2019).

Flax Seed

The seeds and oil of flax seed are rich in omega-3 fatty acids and may be a potent antioxidant and anti-inflammatory. Studies have found that it can help prevent colon cancer, reduce blood pressure, and curb hot flashes. You can harvest the oil, make flour, and eat the seeds with other foods. These seeds can impact estrogen production in women, especially if they are pregnant or have a history of cancer. Raw and unripe seeds can be toxic.

Tea Tree Oil

This plant, native to Australia, has antimicrobial properties in its oil that may be beneficial in treating topical infections, insect bites, minor cuts, mild acne, and athlete's foot. It may negatively impact hormones and can't be orally ingested, and for topical use, be sure to dilute it with a carrier oil before applying it to the skin.

Grapeseed Oil

This antioxidant may lower LDL cholesterol and treat poor circulation in veins and edema. Studies have linked it to anticancer effects. It may reduce iron absorption and the efficacy of pharmaceutical blood thinners and blood pressure medications and should be avoided before surgery.

Ideal Herbs for Detox and Cleansing

Many herbs have been used for centuries to cleanse the body and the mind. Here's a short list of some of my favorites.

Burdock

Burdock is a prickly plant with heart-shaped leaves. The root is used to detox the skin, the blood, and the lymphatic system. It's rich in two powerful antioxidant phenolic acids called quercetin and luteolin, and recent research has found that it can detox heavy metals from the blood, promote blood circulation, and may shrink many cancers. In TCM, it's used to cool down the body, and many ancient cultures have used it as a diuretic. Side effects include dehydration, risk of bleeding during surgery, and allergies. Pregnant women should avoid it, and since this root resembles deadly nightshade, there's a potential risk of contamination. Burdock root products contain the fresh or dried root of the burdock plant. Fresh burdock root can be peeled like a carrot and cooked with food, pickled, and eaten raw, but you should preserve and properly store anything you don't eat within a few days (Price 2024).

Milk Thistle

Milk Thistle is named after the milky white juice produced when its leaves are crushed, and the leaves are also spotted with white. It has long been used as a healing herb that detoxes the blood, liver, and gallbladder from alcohol, heavy metals, pesticides, and airborne pollutants. It's also known to help secrete bile so that we can absorb fat from food. It's also been linked to the prevention of breast cancer and the shrinking of cancer tumors and may also protect against lung and prostate cancer. It may also fight oxidative stress linked to diabetes, heart disease, and neurodegenerative diseases like Alzheimer's and protect the skin from the signs of aging. If you decide to grow milk thistle plants, at harvest, cut off the whole head and hang the plant upside down for about a week; it's easier to collect the seeds. After proper drying, you can eat the seeds raw or make tea by crushing the seeds and steeping them with the leaves. You can also dry the seeds and leaves (Link 2024).

Red Clover

Red clover is another ancient detoxer of the blood, liver, lymphatic system, and skin. The Druids believed it could ward off evil. Indigenous Americans also used it to curb the symptoms of menopause, and they've been validated by modern research, which has found that it's high in phytoestrogens, which may also help with fertility. If you grow these red beauties, harvest while the blooms are still red, not after they turn brown. You can eat fresh red clover raw and dry them to make teas to drink. For skin irritations, you can make a salve or poultice (Timmins Malek 2019).

Energy Boosters and Immune System Powerplants

Here's another short list of my favorite energizing plants and immune system boosters.

Ginseng

Ginseng is a slow-growing plant that can take up to six years to harvest, but it's worth the wait. The Asian variety may boost energy, American ginseng has been found to improve cognitive function, and the Korean red ginseng may boost the immune system. Ginseng is also linked to preventing flu, lowering blood sugar, treating chronic fatigue syndrome, and may even prevent cancer by 16 percent, according to one systematic review. It's not linked to any serious adverse effects, but if you take diabetes medication, talk to your doctor before use (Semeco 2023).

Chia Seeds

Chia seeds are loaded with nutritional value and omega fatty acids that ancient Aztec warriors used to stay energized and alert, and ancient Maya called "strength" and "runner's food." Today, athletes rely on it to boost endurance and build muscle, and its high calcium helps strengthen bones. It's packed with polyphenols, and recent research found that it can stop up to 70 percent of free radical activity. The high-fiber seeds may cause stomach aches if you eat a large portion (Link 2023).

Black Elderberries

Black elderberries are dark purple fruits of the black elder shrub native to Europe. Elderberries have ten times the number of antioxidants as the majority of other berries, and they're high in flavonoids, polyphenols, potassium, and fiber. They're used to treat colds and flu, respiratory issues, and many skin conditions ranging from burns to cancer. Be sure to cook these berries thoroughly before eating or preservation, as they contain a toxin that can cause digestive issues (WebMD 2023).

Echinacea

Echinacea's medicinal powerhouse is the spiky looking cone-headed flower. It may boost immunity to treat colds, viruses, and upper respiratory tract infections. It's generally considered safe to drink in juices and tea, extracts, and supplements (Deering 2019).

Calendula

Calendula petals are bright yellow or orange and look like sunbursts. The flower and the leaves contain many potent antioxidants that neutralize oxidative stress and tumor-killing anti-inflammatory compounds; it's also antimicrobial and antifungal. The extract is used to treat skin wounds, diaper rash, ulcers, and gingivitis, and it may be an ideal natural sunscreen.

Brain Plants for Cognitive Function

Many herbs are ideal for boosting cognitive functions and mood, and others are ideal for soothing the mind, body and spirit. Here are some top contenders:

Sage

Sage has more than 160 powerful plant compounds that improve mood, attention, and memory and treat hot flashes and other symptoms in menopausal women. Animal research has found that it can suppress cancer and stimulate tumor cell death. Sage oil can cause side effects with prolonged use, including nausea, diarrhea, hypertension, and elevated heartbeat, and exposure to the oil is dangerous for young children (Richter 2024).

Gotu Kola

Gotu Kola is also known as the fountain of youth, and scientists have linked it to improving mental clarity, enhancing memory and cognitive skills, increasing blood flow in the brain, and relieving anxiety (Lawler 2023).

Spearmint

Spearmint is another herb that boosts cognitive performance, protects the brain, enhances memory and problem-solving, and may promote the growth of new brain cells. At the same time, it can improve sleep, and you can consume it as a tea or as an extract (Downey 2018).

German Chamomile

German Chamomile has a calming effect that curbs anxiety and insomnia and may provide anticancer benefits. It's been well-studied for safety, even in long-term use, but it may cause allergy-related anaphylaxis and interact with blood thinning medications (Deering 2019).

Now that we know how and why we need to shift to an eco-friendly, sustainable alternative to Big Pharma and Big Food and we have the essential knowledge about key herbal remedies, it's time to put the big "L" into this holistic life plan. In the next chapter, I'll show you how to create a sustainable first aid kit that'll take you even further on the path to a self-sufficient future.

"Look deep into nature, and then you will understand everything better."

- ALBERT EINSTEIN

CHAPTER THREE

Learn About Essential Herbal Remedies

Your First Aid Kit

T he medicine cabinets of our ancient ancestors were just like ours. They had remedies to treat headaches, toothaches, colds and viruses, digestive issues, joint and muscle pain, allergies, and every skin problem, from insect bites and cuts to burns and rashes. The only difference is that theirs had no doors or walls —nature provided their first aid kit.

In this chapter, we'll think outside the modern medicine cabinet box so that you can grow your own herbal remedies and create a first aid kit using the best natural, eco-friendly products.

Aloe

Let's start with *aloe barbadensis*, which ancient Sumerians considered so important that they carved it into their medicinal clay tablets circa 2000 BCE, and soon after, so did the Egyptians (Chelu 2023). Legends suggest that Cleopatra used it as a beauty product, and Alexander the Great captured an island to get his hands on aloe, considering it a must-have to treat his soldiers' battle wounds (Manvitha 2014). Nowadays, most of us know that this spike-leafed plant can soothe sunburns, though it usually comes out of a bottle packed with chemicals and additives, including neon green coloring agents. It's enough to make the ancients turn in their graves. We know that ancient people used aloe to treat headaches, allergies, and ulcers (Aboelsoud 2021). Modern scientists are finally confirming what we've known for thousands of years: that the gel in aloe can treat surface wounds, curb arthritic and rheumatic pain, treat many skin conditions, including psoriasis, treat second degree burns in less than half the time of conventional treatments, and potentially also facilitate burn-related skin grafts; when used internally, it can treat constipation, digestive tract hemorrhoids, and ulcers, and reduce the risk of cardiovascular diseases and cancer. It's also a great cavity-fighting toothpaste, treats mouth ulcers, and promotes stem cell growth in dental pulp (Cronkleton 2018; Chelu 2023).

Aloe is such an effective healing plant that when you cut off a juicy leaf part, the leaf immediately starts to heal itself. It's a prolific grower in any climate and it doesn't need a lot of direct sun or water. The leaves contain a translucent gel that provides so many benefits. Research has found that it contains several active compounds, including acemannan, used in dentistry and pharmaceuticals to treat cardiovascular and tumor-related diseases. Other beneficial ingredients in the gel include potent antiviral, antimicrobial, antifungal, anti-inflammatory, and antidiabetic compounds, along with ingredients that stimulate the production of collagen and new cells and allow DNA synthesis. It contains antioxidant vitamins that neutralize free radicals and improve the absorption of vitamins C and E and enzymes that help optimize the function of the body's metabolic pathways, hormones, and sterols to promote wound healing and antitumor proteins.

With all these incredible ingredients, it's no wonder that aloe has three mechanisms to protect its gel from opportunistic predators: spikes on the leaves; bitter anti-nutrients in the green outer skin of the leaves; and latex, a gummy yellowish liquid that you'll want to extract out of the leaf. Both the leaf skin and latex can cause skin irritation and, if ingested in high amounts, can cause stomach aches and diarrhea; that's why it's used for constipation.

Once I had some latex residue on my fingers when I applied the gel to a sunburn on my face, and some of that latex got into my eye, causing stinging and swelling for a few hours afterwards. It can cause an allergic reaction, including a rash, boils, and blisters (Vialli 2024). Medical studies have found that topical and internal reactions are more common with products that use whole leaf extracts, so the latex could be causing these side effects (Chelu 2023). To ensure safety, follow the steps below to avoid side effects, and ensure that when you apply the gel topically, all of the latex has been drained.

1. Choose a mature leaf, which is one on the lower outside edge of the plant; younger shoots grow closer to the trunk.

2. Wipe off any dust and residue from the leaf.

3. Remove a leaf for use by cutting close to the base of the leaf. You'll see the latex start to leak from the plant. If you're a newbie to fresh aloe, consider removing the leaf's skin with a vegetable peeler. But this step is not necessary as long as you cut the leaf properly so that there's still enough gel inside the green skin.

4. To drain the latex, cut off the plant spikes and place the leaf in a glass with the cut side facing down. It'll take about ten minutes for that yellow liquid to drain into the glass. You'll notice that the latex turns a brownish color as it oxidizes.

5. Remove the leaf from the glass, and if you didn't peel off the green skin, cut the leaf into smaller portions and soak them in a clean glass or bowl for at least eight hours.

6. Wash your hands, scrub under your fingernails, and clean the knife thoroughly to remove any extra latex residue.

7. When you remove a portion of the plant, wipe off any remaining yellow latex from the leaf.

8. Cut through the middle of the leaf portion to expose the fleshy gel.

9. You can apply that gel directly to the skin. But if this is your first time using raw aloe gel, do an allergy test by applying a small amount of the gel to the inside of your arm. Wait twenty-four hours to see if you have an allergic reaction. If not, you can safely apply the gel topically to the skin and hair.

If you don't use the entire leaf with one application, place the remaining leaf part in the fridge in a clean, airtight glass container. You can use the extra portions for approximately one week. You can also freeze the aloe for up to a year, but be sure to put a label on the airtight container with the harvest date (Nunez 2023). Please also read my storage instructions in Chapter Five so that you know how to safely store your herbal remedies to prevent issues like mold and other food safety musts.

Let's look at many other incredible first aid essentials, including treatments for headaches and migraines, toothaches, joint and muscle pain, digestive issues, and skin treatments.

Headaches and Migraines

Feverfew

Feverfew treats headaches and migraines, including side effects like nausea and sensitivity to light and sound. Consuming dried feverfew leaf and extract may be the safest option, though you might have digestive issues. Chewing the raw leaf may cause swelling, mouth sores, and loss of taste (WebMD n.d.).

Willow Bark

Willow bark contains salicin, which is in aspirin, and it may treat colds and flu and muscle pain. It might also slow blot clotting, so don't take it with other blot-clotting drugs or herbal remedies, and as always, don't give it to your children without a doctor's approval (MedlinePlus 2023).

Matcha

Matcha green tea is a great anti-inflammatory that's been shown to treat migraines, headaches, jet lag, alcohol hangovers, and the post-workout crash and burn that many people feel when they use sugary energy drinks. Matcha does contain caffeine, which can also alleviate headaches unless you're sensitive to caffeine (Hadjipateras 2023).

Coriander Seeds

Coriander seeds have been used medically in Persian cultures to treat migraines since the 6th century BCE. Recent medical studies have found that it's significantly better than the standard use of ascorbic acid, and the use of many pharmaceutical drugs to treat migraines often causes many serious side effects. One recent medical study found that after four weeks, 15 ml of coriander was significantly better than placebo at preventing migraines and reducing the frequency and duration. No side effects were observed, though the researchers point out that validation will require long-term follow up and more studies. Coriander is a potent antimicrobial, anti-inflammatory, anticancer, and analgesic (Mansouri 2020).

Toothache Remedies

Garlic

Garlic may cause bad breath, but it's a potent antioxidant and anti-inflammatory, which can reduce pain and swelling. While you're soothing that ache, it's also providing antimicrobial, anti-tumor, and cardiovascular support. Fresh garlic contains more allicin than other preparations, so you can grow garlic and apply a fresh clove directly to the affected area for immediate relief. Be gentle with it; don't push it into the affected area, and use it moderately. Tooth pain could indicate a serious issue, so be sure to see your dentist (Colgate 2024).

Thyme Oil

Thyme Oil has an active analgesic called carvacrol that's known to reduce dental nerve pain. It works best with exposed nerves and might not be effective with unexposed nerves. You can make a mouthwash for use three times a day by mixing one or two drops of thyme oil with one cup of water; swish it around for a minute, spit it out, and rinse with water (Chen 2023).

Joint and Muscle Pain Treatments

I've already mentioned that aloe vera is an effective treatment for joint pain and a great topical quick-fix if you have a supply of prepared aloe in the freezer. Here are two other ideal anti-inflammatory plant-based remedies:

Cayenne Pepper

Cayenne pepper contains capsaicin, which can treat chronic joint pain, including arthritis. Capsaicin can deactivate the natural chronic pain-related signals in the brain, deactivating a hormone linked to chronic pain so that neurotransmitters don't send out that pain alert. It's not a sedative, so you can use it anytime (Khroma 2017). You can make your own capsaicin cream by mixing three tablespoons of powdered cayenne pepper with any organic oil, heating them at medium in a double boiler for ten minutes; add a half cup of grated beeswax until blended, chill in the fridge until cool, stir the mix again, and apply it directly to the painful area. Wash your hands thoroughly; if you touch your eyes while cooking or applying this mix, it can be incredibly irritating. Cayenne can also stain, so put a cloth barrier between your skin and your clothes. Store the rest of the mix in an airtight container in the fridge for up to two weeks. If you don't have pain relief, increase the amount of cayenne pepper, and consider adding two tablespoons of turmeric and two tablespoons of ginger to the mixture since both are potent anti-inflammatories (Everyday Roots 2013).

Borage Seed Oil

Borage seed oil is rich with omega-6 fatty acids, including a high amount of GLA, which helps the joint's function and cell structure by converting the GLA into prostaglandins known to regulate the immune system and fight inflammation. That's ideal for acute injuries, but with chronic inflammation, it's terrible. Clinical trials have shown it can effectively treat rheumatoid arthritis, but scientists require more validation. Always check with your doctor first, especially if you take blood thinners or have liver diseases (Herbaugh 2021).

Herbal Digestive Tract Remedies

Many of us know that ginger is a great anti-nausea treatment because we were given ginger ale to treat stomach aches and motion sickness. I've already discussed the many benefits of ginger, which you can chew raw or add to tea to soothe your belly and so much more. Here are two more herbs that can treat indigestion, constipation, diarrhea, and other digestive tract conditions.

Licorice Root

Licorice root is a digestive tract powerhouse with a long history of use in TCM and Ayurveda; the ancient Greeks called it "sweet root." Modern research has confirmed it may be a great bellyache reliever and an ideal acid reflux treatment, with the added benefit of increased mucus that protects the esophagus from acidic damage. Side effects include increased blood pressure, so if you have cardiovascular conditions or any health-related issues, always ask your doctor first (McGaha 2024).

Fennel

Fennel is a tall drink of goodness. This big, antioxidant-rich plant can grow up to eight feet tall, and you can eat all of it, from its feathery fronds to its bulging bulb. In many cultures, fennel is still eaten at the end of a meal as a gas-preventing digestive aid. It can also relieve period cramps and soothe colic in babies, but ask your doctor first, please. You can eat it raw or in cooked foods, dry it to make tea, or create fennel-spiked oil (Braverman 2024).

Bites, Stings, Wounds, Burns, and Skin Irritations

I've already mentioned calendula as a great option to use as a sunscreen and to treat wounds, diaper rash, ulcers, and gingivitis. Lavender, also mentioned earlier, is another ideal plant for treating skin conditions and anxiety. Here are two more essentials for your first aid kit:

Yarrow

Yarrow was found in the dental plaque of the fifty-thousand-year-old Neanderthal we met in the first chapter. This perennial flowering plant is also a star of the "Achilles Heel" legend. The story goes that when this

Greek demigod was just a babe, his mom dipped him in a yarrow bath to protect him from harm, but she missed a heel. The mistake caught up with him when he became a soldier, and an arrow pierced the sensitive spot on his heel. Yarrow is an ideal antiseptic, antibacterial, anti-fungal, astringent, anti-inflammatory herb. It's known to stop cuts from bleeding and can disinfect skin wounds, treat insect bites and stings, and ease headaches, toothaches, colds and flu, and menstrual cramps. If you're in a pinch, you can apply the leaves directly to the skin, or you can dry the stems, leaves, and flowers to make teas, tinctures, and poultices (Potter 2015.).

Comfrey

Comfrey is a tall shrub with bell-shaped flowers that's been a staple in Japan for more than two thousand years. It's also known as "knit bone," and recent medical research has confirmed it may be useful to treat injuries like ankle sprains, osteoarthritis, and back pain. Topical applications on unbroken skin appear safe, but it's not recommended for oral use because it contains alkaloids linked to cancer, severe liver damage, and death (Goldman 2017).

Marshmallow Root

Marshmallow root contains a sap-like, sticky, gelatinous substance that rehydrates and protects the skin, making it ideal for abrasions, bites, and many skin conditions, including allergies and eczema. Animal studies have also shown that it provides UV protection and may heal sun-damaged skin. It's also effective with colds and flu, bacterial infections in the bladder and urinary tract, and inflammatory joint pain and IBS. I'm not surprised Homer mentioned this "slippery" herb in *The Iliad*, his epic poem about the Trojan War. It's generally considered safe, but this sticky substance can interact with the absorption of medications. You can dry or freeze the root and the leaves and make excellent salves and teas (Levy 2021).

Allergy Relieving Herbs

Stinging Nettle

Stinging nettle is named after the stinging sensation you get when you brush up against this plant's hairy stem and leaves, but it has a soothing effect with treating hay fever and allergy symptoms and may also speed up wound healing. The leaves need to be cooked to destroy the hairy covering, which can cause itchy rashes—something you certainly want to avoid when treating allergies (Metcalf 2023).

Butterbur

Butterbur is a perennial shrub with large, round leaves, named for its traditional use as a wrap for butter to protect against melting. It has long been used to treat asthma, coughs, migraines, and seasonal allergies like hay fever, thanks to petacins, highly concentrated in the plant's roots, that have antihistamine and anti-inflammatory properties. It's also a rich source of flavonoids, tannins, and sesquiterpenes that, like petacins, inhibit the body's inflammatory response by blocking the effect of histamines. Please note that raw butterbur can be toxic to the liver, so you need to cook or dry the root and store it properly to make teas and oils, which I'll show you how to do in Chapter Five (Atkins 2023).

Lean Into Nature

Now that you have some ideal herbal options for your medicine cabinet, you can lean on ancient wisdom and nature's abundant riches to treat your first-aid needs. Once your garden is producing effective organic herbs and plants, which we'll dig into in Chapter 5, I'll show you how to make herbal remedies, personal products, and household cleaning supplies so that you have organic, sustainable, healthy and effective. You'll be much more self-sufficient when you need it most, and you won't need to run to the pharmacy and supermarket to buy environmentally unfriendly products that are often less effective and contain many unnecessary synthetic chemicals linked to many side effects.

First, let's take a deeper look into the most common diseases and chronic conditions linked to disability and mortality and talk about the optimal herbs for prevention, treatment, and lifelong health and longevity. By the time you finish this next chapter, you'll have all the essential knowledge to choose the ideal plants for you, and you'll be ready for my step-by-step guide to creating your own sustainable garden.

"The cure of many diseases is unknown to physicians... because they are ignorant of the whole. For the part can never be well unless the whole is well."

— PLATO

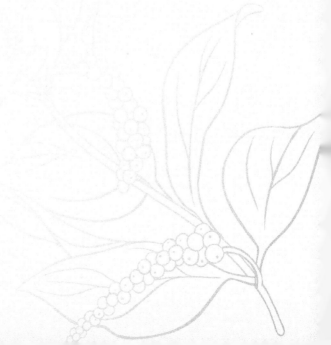

CHAPTER FOUR

Invigorate Your Health with Phytonutrient-Loaded Plants

Treat the Top Diseases and Chronic Conditions

H ave you ever faced a health crisis and felt like you'd never become healthy and whole again? Like your body—and the world—was out to get you? After my gallbladder was removed and I was waiting for medical test results to find out why I had painful digestive issues, I felt like I was trapped in my own body and alienated from the world around me; it seemed to reflect and echo my own health crisis, and I had the sense that everything was out of balance and headed to catastrophe. At first, I couldn't see a way out of it. Luckily, I had a lot of support from my family, especially my partner, who opened the door to the world of sustainable, eco-friendly herbal medicine. It fortified my strength—my roots in the natural world—and gave me the confidence to do so much more than simply manage my health issues and survive; it gave me the wisdom, skills, motivation, and confidence to become self-empowered, heal, and thrive.

In this chapter, we'll explore this alternate world that, for many of us, has been hiding in plain sight all along. We'll focus on the diseases and conditions most likely to cause health issues and mortality: cardiovascular diseases, cancers, respiratory illnesses, autoimmune conditions, and neurological, aging-related diseases. For each section, I'll provide information about potent plant-based herbal remedies scientifically linked to prevention and treatment, with a focus on fresh and dried plants that you can grow and enjoy straight from the garden. Please take note that if you currently have one of these conditions and you're taking pharmaceutical therapies to treat any condition or plan to have surgery, it's imperative to talk to your doctor and do some research for yourself about contraindications. Even if you're eating these plants, that's the safest way to enjoy the health benefits, especially for healthy people looking for preventative options.

Heart Health

Fruits and veggies known to lower blood pressure include berries, citrus fruits, bananas, avocados, beets, tomatoes, spinach, Swiss chard, carrots, celery, and broccoli, and seeds such as chia and flaxseed (Leonard 2024).

Garlic

Garlic is packed with powerful antioxidants, including selenium, vitamin C, manganese, and quercetin, a potent phytonutrient anti-inflammatory. This member of the onion family can fight high blood pressure, a condition that nearly half of Americans have. Analysis of twelve clinical studies found that garlic supplements lower blood pressure, reducing the risk of cardiovascular disease by up to 40 percent. It's also linked to helping prevent atherosclerosis (hardening of the arteries), and another review of studies done from the 1950s until 2013 found that this ancient crop can "moderately to significantly" lower total cholesterol levels, including LDL, known as the "bad" cholesterol.

With at least 184 bioactive compounds, including polysaccharides, saponins, tannins, phenols, amino acids and the highest amount of allicin (an organosulfur compound) in its family of plants, allicin comprises up to 80 percent of garlic's bioactive compounds, and consuming raw garlic is the ideal way to benefit. There's good research evidence that garlic is an antihypertensive, cardioprotective, antithrombotic, anticarcinogenic, antidiabetic, anti-obesity and anticancer, including of the lung, gastrointestinal, and urinary tract. Much of the good stuff is in the bulb, but the leaf also has antioxidant and anti-inflammatory compounds (Mohamed 2024). Research has confirmed that we can benefit from these potent biocompounds by eating garlic, but you can also take it as an extract. Suggested doses are four grams of fresh garlic, 7.5 grams of "aged" garlic extract, or a dried garlic powder tablet up to four times per day. Be sure to avoid consuming raw garlic (or any supplement) on an empty stomach, which can cause digestive issues and even tachycardia (Mohamed 2024).

Parsley

Parsley is an aromatic staple of the Mediterranean diet. It comes in two types, curly leaf (aka French) and flat leaf (aka Italian). It's known to reduce blood pressure, in part because it's a rich source of apigenin, a flavonoid linked to preventing initial arteriosclerosis in cells and reducing the effects of vascular inflammation (Yamagata 2019). It also reduces myocardial ischemia, the cardiovascular impact of type 2 diabetes, hypertension and drug-induced cardiotoxicity, and has anticancer, chemo preventative, and chemotherapeutic benefits, too (Turner 2023). Dried parsley is the best natural source of apigenin, and flavones are also in the flowers. Parsley (and celery and oregano, two other great apigenin sources) is linked to many cardioprotective effects. It's also rich in vitamin K; a single tablespoon of fresh parsley provides more than 70 percent of the recommended daily intake (WebMD 2022), with 215 ml of apogenin in fresh parsley and more than forty-five thousand in dried parsley. There are few clinical reports of apigenin-related adverse effects, though researchers acknowledge more research is required to establish safety parameters (Turner 2023). Meanwhile, enjoy fresh or dried parsley in your food and as an ideal garnish.

Basil

Basil is a staple in ancient herbal medicine. It's a great free radical fighter, reducing the risk of heart disease, cancer, diabetes, and arthritis. There are more than sixty types of basil, including the most common, sweet basil (which contains eugenol, ideal for lowering blood pressure and cholesterol); lime and lemon (which contains limonene, an anti-inflammatory); and holy basil (which research has linked with improved immunity and decreased asthma-related airway swelling, stress, anxiety, and depression. That's no surprise to Ayurveda practitioners, since they emphasize the mind-body-spirit balance and rely on the holy basil plant for health, worship, prayer, and spiritual rituals. The Ancient Greeks loved it, too, and gave it the Latin name for "royal." Basil is rich in antioxidants, but the potency diminishes significantly during the drying process, so choose fresh basil, and if you add it to your cooked food, toss some into your recipe near or at the end because it contains volatile oils that diminish flavor. No safety issues are linked to basil, but as always, check with your doctor if you have a disease or are taking medications. (WebMd 2023).

Cardamom

Cardamom is a prized aromatic spice in TCM. Known as the queen of spices in Ayurvedic medicine, it's used to eliminate toxins and aid diges-tion. It's also one of the most expensive spices after vanilla and saffron (Ayurveda Living), which I'll discuss in the next section. Cardamom be-longs to the same plant family as ginger. Its medicinal benefit is in the seed pods, which can be ground into powder and used for both sweet and sa-vory dishes. It might also treat heart diseases; a systematic review of carda-mom supplements found it could significantly lower triglyceride levels that cause plague in blood vessels and increase risk of stroke, heart attack, and heart diseases. In another small study of twenty people, a half teaspoon per day for twelve weeks reduced blood pressure. It's also shown promise with lowering blood sugar in people with type 2 diabetes and decreasing liver inflammation; preclinical research suggested it may reduce cancer apoptosis. It's not FDA-approved for any conditions, but clinical studies on people used on 1.5-6 grams per day (Barnes 2022). It can take two years for this plant to bear seed pods for medicinal use, but if you're patient, and you live in a climate with an average temperature between ten and thirty-five degrees Celsius and you also get plenty of rainfall, give it a try (Kumari 2022).

Cancer Prevention, Treatments, and Adjuvants

According the latest data, there were twenty million new cases of cancer in 2022 and 9.7 million cancer deaths. About one in five people get cancer at some point in their lives; one in nine men and one in twelve women will die from it. Lung cancer was the most frequently diagnosed type, and had the highest mortality, followed by colorectal, breast, and stomach cancer. By 2050, predictions indicate thirty-five million new cancer cases (Bray et al. 2024).

We've already discussed the potential anticancer benefits of ginger, ginseng, garlic, turmeric, ginkgo flax seed, milk thistle, aloe vera, and many other plants. These plant-based compounds are currently being used to prevent and treat cancer, help reduce the side effects of conventional cancer treatments, and as an adjuvant that have been found to help prevent cancer from returning. I mentioned earlier that medical scientists have identified more than six hundred anticancer plant compounds, which account for 50 percent of all anticancer agents, yet only 10 percent have been investigated for pharmaceutical use (Muhammad 2022). Researchers at the US National Institute of Health recently documented that among the 1,881 approved new drugs of the past four decades, 929 had a natural origin (Dehelean et al. 2021), classified as "natural," "natural product botanical," and "natural product mimics" (Newman & Cragg 2020), including 240 antitumor drugs, and only twenty-nine are strictly synthetic drugs (Dehelean et al. 2021).

Key plants and natural compounds with known anticancer properties include (Dehelean et al. 2021):

- Curcumin

- Ginseng

- Resveratrol (found in grapes, peanuts, cranberries and blueberries)

- Quercetin, compounds containing artemisinin (found in *Artemisia annua*, also known as annual mugwort, annual wormwood, and sweet sagewort)

- Apigenin compounds (found in *Lycopodium clavatum*, also known as common club moss and stag's horn clubmoss*)*

- Parsley (Petroselinum crispum)

- Celery (Apium graveolens)

- Luteolin flavones, (found in *Salvia tomentosa*, AKA balsamic sage)

- Genistein (an isoflavone and natural dietary polyphenol commonly found in soybean)

Shitake Mushrooms

Shitake mushrooms are also showing a lot of promise in treating cancer and providing relief from chemotherapy treatments. This mushroom is native to East Asia, is a common ingredient in Asian cooking, and, according to conventional cancer research, a potent anticancer remedy. Some of the active medicinal compounds include lentinan, a polysaccharide with immunostimulatory, hepatoprotective, antiviral, cytotoxic, and antimutagenic capabilities. Preclinical research also found that dried shiitake extract caused apoptosis in human hepatocellular carcinoma (HepG2) cells and inhibited lung cancer cells, leading to apoptotic induction. It appears to have the ability to suppress enzymes known to metabolize procarcinogens to active forms, and other polysaccharides also had antitumor effects, inducing apoptosis in tumor cells in mice. Clinical research involving patients with advanced gastrointestinal cancer found that oral shiitake mycelial extract decreased the incidence of chemotherapy-associated adverse effects and improved quality of life. Other research among adults that eat shitake mushrooms found it improved immune function via increased proliferation tumor necrosis factor (TNF)-α levels.

Potential side effects include skin inflammation, elevated white blood cell levels, stomachache, and spore-sensitivity related hypersensitivity (MSKCC 2023).

Respiratory and Lung Health

Many herbs benefit the lungs and respiratory system as expectorants and antitussives (to break up mucus and reduce coughing), respiratory demulcents that reduce inflammation and soothe the respiratory system, spasmolytics that relax airway muscles, and antiallergic compounds. Here are some ideal herbal options to treat respiratory disorders (Powers 2022):

- ▸ **Horehound** is a great expectorant, approved by the European Medicines Agency (EMA).

- ▸ **Stinging nettle** may provide relief from seasonal allergies; clinical studies found it was better than placebo and reduced allergic rhinitis.

- ▸ **Mullein** is a longtime favorite of herbalists as an expectorant, reducing inflammation. It contains many anti-inflammatories and antioxidants

- ▸ **Eyebright** is another EMA-approved herbal medicine to treat cold symptoms, and the American Botanical Council recommends it for fevers, cough, sore throat and earaches.

Autoimmune Conditions

Boswellia

Boswellia, also known as Indian Frankincense, has been scientifically linked to reducing inflammation and may be useful for osteoarthritis and rheumatoid arthritis (and related joint pain and swelling), inflammatory bowel disease, Crohn's disease, and asthma. The medicinal value is in the plant's resin. Pregnant women should avoid this plant as it may cause nausea, skin rash, and diarrhea (Moncivaiz 2018).

Saffron

Saffron is a favorite in ancient herbal medicine, and it's the most expensive spice in the world. To make one pound of the spice, you'll need up to 125,000 flowers because the medicinal part is in the three stigmas inside each blooming flower. Saffron flowers only live for two days max, so come fall harvest, you'll need to get up early to get the stigmas as soon as you see them. But this perennial is easy to grow if you have a sunny spot and well-draining soil. Use tweezers to pluck the stigmas and put them in a well-ventilated dark spot to dry for up to five days before you store them in an airtight container. Properly stored, they can last up to two years. The Romans used saffron to treat upper respiratory tract infections, and in Ayervedic medicine, it's an expectorant and anti-asthma. Modern research has found 150 compounds in saffron's red stigmas, which may provide anticancer, anti-inflammatory, antioxidant, anti-allergic, anti-diabetic, anti-obesity, neuroprotective, cardioprotective, and antidepressant benefits. Avoid taking it therapeutically if you're pregnant or plan to be soon; it can also cause nausea, headache, and serious side effects if taken in high doses (Price 2023).

Natural Remedies for Alzheimer s and Dementia

Many of us have already seen our parents or grandparents experience the debilitating effects of dementia and Alzheimer's. So far, conventional medicine has found no medications that can prevent or cure these diseases and few that might slow the progress of cognitive decline, though they tend to come with other side effects. Evidence so far suggests that lifestyle factors might help, including following a heart-healthy diet, exercising regularly, and maintaining an active social life (Mayo Clinic 2024).

Medical research on plant-based treatment options to improve cognitive function has focused on the ideal antioxidant, anti-inflammatory, adaptogenic and neuroprotective compounds linked to brain health. Adaptogenic herbs relieve mental stress by decreasing cortisol levels. Chronic stress imbalances the hypothalamic–pituitary–adrenal axis, causing elevated cortisol levels, linked to a variety of ailments and diseases related to cognitive impairment, including memory loss. Academic researchers recently published a paper about nine adaptogenic herbs, analyzing twenty-five studies, and noted that chronic psychological stress can be "the breeding ground" for many diseases and disorders, including cardio-vascular, cognitive impairment, and mental disorders (Tóth-Mészáros 2023). They looked at many herbs linked to improved cognitive function and physical and mental endurance, including *eleutherococcus senticosis*, commonly known as Siberian ginseng or devil's bush. The researchers concluded that *withania somnifera* (ashwagandha root, also known as winter cherry), a member of the nightshade family, decreases decreased cortisol and stress levels among healthy adults, with only minor, transitory side effects, though more research will be required among people with cognitive disorders.

Resources for Seeking Ideal Plants and Herbal Remedies.

I know that it can be incredibly challenging to research a specific health disorder while you're in the midst of dealing with the debilitating side effects. You need to research the medications that the doctors recommend and look at their benefits, risks, side effects, and all the food and plants that may be contraindicated. Drugs.com provides comprehensive lists of drugs and contraindications, and this book's reference list includes links to key resources, including published medical literature, and articles from medical writers, also medically reviewed by doctors. As I mentioned earlier, PubMed is also a great resource for researching plant and herbal remedies for specific conditions and diseases.

As I keep saying, it's imperative to talk to your doctor before using these herbal remedies, but not all doctors and specialists are trained in food-based, plant-based herbal remedies. You could consider consulting with a certified naturopath that specializes in natural remedies. I also recommend consulting a herbal medicine practitioner, but in the US, there is no federally recognized licensing agency for herbal medicine, and according to the Herbal Academy (Herbal Academy n.d.), it's illegal for herbalists to "treat, cure, or prescribe" because they're not licensed, so any individual or school that claims to be "certified," or calls themselves a "master" in herbal remedies is "stretching the truth."

I highly recommend that you pace yourself with this complex research. Choose one health condition and dive into the science and the ancient history of these plants and herbs. As I said earlier, if you're healthy, it's usually safe to eat or drink a moderate amount of plants and herbs as part of your daily diet, and if you want to start increasing the amount or using a potent herbal remedy, start with a low dose and watch for side effects. But if you've been diagnosed with a specific disease or condition, you're taking medications, you're pregnant or breastfeeding, or you want to provide medicinal herbs to children, you will need to do your research and rely on medical support.

I don't want to demotivate you from becoming self-empowered and self-sufficient—I want you to be rooted, balanced and eager to explore the world of plant-based remedies. I think the best way to do that is to start your own garden. It helped me immensely because I started reconnecting with nature, and when I did that, I wanted to live and thrive, and I wanted everything in the natural world to thrive, too. But I also did a ton of scientific research before I chose the plants and herbs I wanted to cultivate and make into home remedies. I hope the research provided so far in this book is a jumping off point for you to do your own research and customize your garden to your personal goals, whether these goals are preventative, therapeutic, or about making your life more sustainable and future-proof.

In the next chapter, I'll show you how to create a sustainable, eco-friendly herb garden, how to harvest and store your herbals, and how to isolate potent plant parts so that you can make herbal remedies, including infusions, tinctures, and salves. Let's start growing and evolving by creating a garden of earthly delights.

"Adopt the power of nature: her secret is patience."

– RALPH WALDO EMERSON

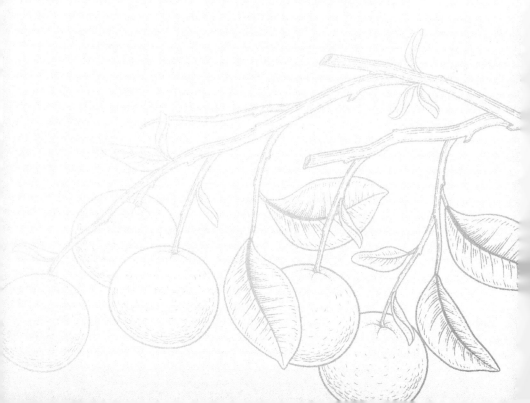

CHAPTER FIVE

The Step-By-Step Guide to Creating Your Own Herb Garden

Sustainable and eco-friendly Indoor Herb Garden

N ow that you have some knowledge of the key plants and herbs that can supercharge your health and well-being and fill your medicine cabinet, you're almost ready to say goodbye to store-bought herbs in plastic wrap or dried spices in plastic containers and bags. You can grow an eco-friendly, sustainable indoor herb garden, even if you don't have a lot of space and money. We'll start with the essential equipment you'll need to get started so that you can grow, care for, harvest, and store your plant parts and enjoy medicinal plants year-round. I'll take you through a step-by-step guide and show you how to turn your harvested and preserved herbal medicines into infusions, poultices, salves, creams, and syrups so that you have a great variety of remedies.

Many of us don't have the time or the space to cultivate a fruit and vege-table garden. But we can have a great year-round indoor herb garden, even in the smallest home. For all of your other needs, I encourage you to limit or stop relying on the Big Food conglomerates and shift your support to local organic farms. Once your herb garden is thriving and you've learned how to make herbal medicines, you could sell or trade your produce with other organic farmers in your community. You'll enjoy fantastic organic food and incredible herbal remedies, forge new connections in your community, and protect the planet. Let's get started!

Choosing Your Seeds

Start by identifying the plants that you want to grow for your pantry and for herbal remedies. Think about your specific health and wellness needs and choose a selection of plants known to have optimal impact on specific aspects of health, including preventative and therapeutic options and essential first aid ingredients for your medicine cabinet. In the next chapter, I'll provide additional suggestions for mental health and wellness, so if these health care options fit your immediate needs, please look through that chapter, too.

Buy only certified organic seeds, ideally 100 percent certified organic. I highly recommend getting your seeds from a local farm. If that's not possible, here are a few links:

▸ If you live in the US, here are three options for organic seeds: https://backtotheroots.com/ ; https://www.trueleafmarket.com/ ; https://www.theorganicharvest.com/

▸ If you live in Canada, check out this list from the Canadian Organic Growers: https://cog.ca/organic-seed-directory/

▸ If you live in the UK, try: https://www.realseeds.co.uk/

Herb Garden Basics

You don't need a lot of equipment or space to create an eco-friendly indoor herbal garden, particularly during the initial seed starter stage.

▸ An indoor space is ideal for starting seeds because young plants can grow in a stable environment, free from the risk of cold, extreme heat and wind, rain, or damp conditions that could cause rot, pests, and diseases (Almanac 2024a).

▸ At this initial stage, your seedlings will need at least six hours of southern sunlight, ideally ten to thirteen hours of sunlight. A south-facing windowsill is an ideal spot, or if you want to grow many herbs and have a large, south-facing window, you could use a vertical shelf that's shaped like a stepladder so that all your herbs get the required sunlight. If that's not doable or you're starting your seedling garden during the short days of winter, you'll need LED or fluorescent grow lights.

▸ You can grow seeds outdoors as long as the low nightly temperature doesn't reach frost level, daytime highs aren't extreme, and your seedlings aren't exposed to a lot of wind.

▸ For an outdoor herb seedling garden, consider creating a raised garden bed with an enclosure to help control weather conditions.

▸ The Old Farmer's Almanac has a useful planting calendar that you can customize to your location in the US and Canada, and it includes ideal planting dates for many plants (Almanac 2024b).

▸ Another advantage of an indoor seedling garden is that you can get started in the winter, especially if you're in a region with a short growing season.

Annual and Perennial Plants

Another factor to consider before you get started is whether your herbs are annual or perennial. Annuals have only one season, and they typically don't like cold weather, so you'll need to replant them every year. Popular annual herbs include German chamomile, basil, fennel, and parsley. Perennials will come back for many seasons, though some perennials are more tender than others and don't tolerate cold, so if you live in a cold climate, you may need to plant new ones or bring them inside during winter. Popular perennial herbs include lavender, mint, sage, and feverfew (Risenmay, n.d.). Once your herbs are in containers or in the soil, many require full sunlight, but some can tolerate partial shade. If you're getting seeds from an organic seed provider, the packaging should include the type of seed and tips for ideal planting conditions.

Equipment for Your Indoor Herb Garden

▶ Eco-friendly seed starter cups or starter trays

▶ Cover mats

▶ A tray to place under the cups or starter trays

▶ Plant labels

▶ An organic seed starter mix

▶ A watering can and sprayer

▶ A space that provides ten to thirteen hours of western or southern sunlight.

▶ Containers for transplanted plants or an outdoor space for your herb garden

> An organic soil mix and organic fertilizer, ideally made from composted earth

> Scissors or small pruning shears

You can also buy kits with all the necessary equipment for growing seedlings, including attached, extendable lights that can be customized to the growth of your seedlings. Check out this guide by The Spruce: https://www.thespruce.com/best-grow-lights-4158720. But if you have enough sunlight, I prefer the DIY approach. Let's get started with a step-by-step guide to setting up your indoor garden.

A Step-By-Step Herb Garden Starter Guide

The initial seedling starter phase should take approximately ten weeks. After that, you'll transplant the plants to soil-based containers.

1. Choose non-plastic seed starter trays that are about 4 inches deep and provide drainage. Paper-based egg cartons, toilet paper rolls, and cover mats made from biodegradable plastic bags are ideal DIY starter trays because they're economical, biodegradable, and eco-friendly. A bonus is that egg carton cups can be transplanted directly into containers once your seedlings are ready for soil. Make sure that your egg carton is clean, dry, and mold-free at the start. Throughout the stages of growth, be sure not to overwater because paper-based cups don't have drain holes, and seedlings require air circulation, so remove the cover when the seeds begin to germinate (Hodge 2023).

2. Make individual cups for each herb with the egg carton. This provides space for each seedling to grow and makes it easier to transfer your seedlings into larger containers later.

3. Label each cup with the herb name and the planting date, and place the label just below the container's top rim.

4. Make a starter mix; you don't need soil at this stage. You can get these ingredients at your local garden center: perlite, vermiculite, and either sphagnum peat moss or coco coir. Mix equal parts of each of the three ingredients (Ly 2011).

5. Moisten the starter mix with a little water so that the mix has the moisture of a squeezed sponge.

6. Place the mix in each cup and fill to the top. Avoid packing this starter mix too much because initial root growth requires the soil to be light and fluffy.

7. In each cup, create a hole in the middle of the starter mix at a depth that's approximately twice the size of the seed and three times the width of the seed. You can use your finger or a pencil to make this hole.

8. Drop five seeds in the hole and cover it with the starter mix. Give the mix a light spray of water, just enough to give the seed a little moisture.

9. Place the cups on a tray and cover the cups with biodegradable plastic. This cover mat will help keep your plants warm and the conditions slightly humid to speed up the germination period and keep the mix consistently moist.

10. Place the cups on a windowsill that provides at least ten hours of western or southern exposure. Your seedlings will also need a temperature of between 65-75°F. If you don't have any sunlit spaces, use grow lights or fluorescent lights and position the light about three to four inches above the seedling tray.

11. Moisten the seedlings twice weekly with a light sprinkle or spray of water. To prevent overwatering, which can cause a fungal disease that can kill your seedlings and attract fungal gnats, add moisture when the starter mix has become slightly dry.

12. Each time you moisturize your seedlings, rotate the cups so that all sides of the cup receive equal exposure to sunlight. As the days and weeks pass, they'll require more water.

13. Monitor the seedlings for insects, dry soil, and mold, and if mold does appear, place the container in a place that gets more air circulation.

14. For the next six to eight weeks, monitor the plant's growth. When you see sprouts, remove the cover mat.

15. If the weather permits, start exposing the seeds to an hour of outdoor sunlight and moderate wind. Every few days, increase the amount of time they spend outdoors, which reduces the risk of transplant shock. If you can't provide your plants with some outdoor time, use a fan on a low setting to simulate wind, which stimulates auxin, a hormone that strengthens the stem.

16. Within six to eight weeks, the plant should develop into a bushy plant, not a leggy, "stretched" plant. Your plant shouldn't be wilted (which may indicate it's overwatered or underwatered) or crispy with yellow edges (indicating too much exposure to heat and sunlight). If the plant becomes too leggy or any sprouts show signs of damage, remove these sprouts by gently pinching them off or clipping them with scissors.

17. At ten weeks, your plants should be approximately three to four inches high and "hardened off" enough to transplant the seedlings

into a soil-based container. If there are multiple plants in the cup, choose the healthiest plant for transplant. If you're in a warm climate with lots of sunlight, you can plant them in soil with at least six hours of sunlight exposure, though some plants require more or less sunlight. Some herbs can be planted outside in early spring, and for other herbs, you'll need to wait until late spring when there's no risk of frost. The University of Illinois has a great website providing details about the ideal weather conditions and growing tips for a wide assortment of annual and perennial plants. Check it out here: https://extension.illinois.edu/herbs

18. "Hardened off" means your plant has had time to acclimate to fluctuating lighting conditions and temperatures. If you're planting your herbs outside, the wind is another factor that can endanger herbs that haven't had time to acclimate to outdoor conditions.

19. A hardy root is the key factor for transplant. To know if it's ready for transplant, it should be strong enough that when you gently squeeze the sides of the cup, the plant root and the starter mix are one unit, and the mix doesn't fall away from the root.

Container Transplant Guide

The ideal container should be made of natural materials, like cedar or terra cotta. They need drainage holes at the bottom, spaced three to four inches apart, and should be sized two to three inches wider and deeper than the egg cup. A general rule of thumb is a container depth of six inches, but herbs with a larger root tap may need a deeper container.

1. Line the bottom of the container with burlap or an organic landscape cloth so that the container can breathe but doesn't leak soil.

For herbs that like dry conditions, place a layer of sand above the cloth.

2. Fill the container with organic potting soil, leaving about one inch of space at the top. Dig a hole in the soil.

3. Gently remove the plant from the cup, place it in the hole, and gently press the soil around the plant base.

4. Gradually water the plant until the soil is moist but not overwatered. Water every three days or whenever the soil is dry to the touch.

5. Your herbs will need fertilizer at least once per month and whenever they show signs of wilt, so be sure to use an organic fertilizer; you can make your own with the recipe provided in the section below called "Eco-friendly Tips."

6. If you're transplanting your young herbs to outdoor soil, follow the same directions as above. Before digging the hole, till the soil to loosen it up and remove weeds that could choke your plant.

7. Prune your plants at least once monthly to keep their growth productive and prevent your plants from going to seed. For herbal remedies that use the flower of the plant and other plant parts, keep some plants well-pruned and let other plants bloom.

8. Long term, your perennial herbs will need to be divided. Give them a little water before removing them from the container or soil, then divide them by cutting down the middle of the root system. Replant the two halves in separate containers or areas of outdoor soil (Svedi 2021).

Companion Plants

"Companion planting" a few herbs in the same container or outdoor garden is a great way to save space, and plants love all the perks. Companion planting helps repel insects and pests and attract ideal pollinators, like honeybees. They also amplify the amount of nutrients in the soil, release chemicals that boost plant growth, and even improve the flavor and aroma of the herbs. Be sure to avoid pairing up herbs that tend to spread rapidly and choke other roots or herbs that have very specific aromas and flavors, like various mint herbs, which will lose their distinct traits. Good companion plants require the same soil type, amount of water, and sunlight exposure requirements. The goal is to mix plants that thrive in specific regions and mimic these conditions in your indoor or outdoor garden (Stankiewicz 2022).

Eco-friendly Tips

There are many ways you can add layers of environmental friendliness to your gardening practices.

▸ Collect rainwater and reuse water from leftover cooking, like from rice, pasta, and vegetables; this cooking water contains beneficial nutrients as long as there's no salt in the water. Make sure the water has cooled to room temperature before watering your plants.

▸ Make a fertilizer with a combination of one gallon of reused water mixed with your food scraps, including one cup of crushed eggshells, one tablespoon of coffee grounds, a few green tea bags, and a few banana peels. After seeping this mix together for at least an hour, remove the banana peels and water your plants with this organic plant food mix (Jerez Torres 2022).

Composting

You can also make your own organic soil by composting your gardening and food scraps. An ideal compost is a mix of "brown" carbon-rich and "green" nitrogen-rich scraps. Brown scraps include dry leaves and twigs, plant stalks, and shredded paper that's unbleached, nonglossy, and uncolored; green materials include fruit and vegetables scraps, coffee grounds and paper filters, unstapled paper tea bags, and crushed eggshells. Don't compost anything that contains pesticides, herbicides, weeds, or any nonorganic products. If you have big scraps, like pineapple husks and corncobs, break them down into small pieces to speed up the composting process.

You'll want the base of the compost to contain browns, and then you can layer it with greens and browns. The mix should be a ratio of three parts brown to one part green. Aerate the compost by turning it as often as possible and add moisture so that your compost is the consistency of a sponge. To avoid attracting pests, you'll need a compost bin with a solid lid and many small aeration holes on all sides, with no holes larger than one-quarter inch. You'll know the compost is almost ready when you can't see any food scraps and the pile is no longer letting off heat. Let it cure for a month until it shrinks by two-thirds and looks and smells like fresh soil. If you're following all the tips provided above, the entire process will take three to five months (EPA 2024).

Harvesting Your Plants

The ideal time to harvest is on a sunny morning, once the dew evaporates and before the harsh midday sun. Ideal harvesting conditions and methods vary depending on the plant part you want to use (Groves 2019).

1. Start by discarding all the stems and plant parts that are discolored, damaged, or bruised.

2. To harvest leaves and stems that branch from a main stem, focus on the top two-thirds of the plant, and if the plant is a perennial, leave some leaves behind for the next harvest. Cut stems above a leaf node so that the stem will grow back.

3. If the plant has no branch system, like chives and lemongrass, cut a part of the plant right to the soil but leave at least one-third of the plant for the next harvest.

4. If you're not using the flower seeds or flower parts, flowering herbs should have buds but not full blossoms. Pinch off the bud from the lower base and leave the entire bud intact.

5. If you're harvesting seeds and flower parts, wait until the flower has bloomed.

6. Bark is often harvested in spring when the sap is ideal but the tree isn't full of leaves, though you can harvest many barks all year round. Don't harvest from the tree trunk; choose bark from the branches and cut above a strong branch node to encourage new growth or just above the trunk. With younger branches of approximately one and a half inches, you don't need to remove the outer bark, but that's necessary with mature, wide branches. You can remove the bark with a knife or a vegetable peeler.

7. For root harvesting, use a garden fork or digging stick to get to the root and then remove a part of the root crown with a sharp knife or spade. Scrub any soil and debris from the root and clean the root in cold water. Ideally, roots are processed when fresh.

Storage Preparation

After harvesting, you'll need to choose a storage preparation method; some herbs are ideal with the drying technique and others with freezing (Boyle 2023).

Drying Techniques

To effectively dry your herbs, you'll need to start with some heat, humidity, and air circulation. You can buy a food dehydrator or use one of the following methods.

The traditional method is to tie the stems together and hang the herbs from the stems. Start by rinsing the herbs in water and then begin the drying process by leaving them in the sun for a few hours. After that, the ideal place to finish the drying process is a warm, dry, ventilated spot. It'll take one to two weeks for herbs to dry, depending on the climate. They must be totally dry to prevent mold (Herman 2021). Once they're dry and can crumble and flake, remove the leaves from the stems and follow one of the pasteurization methods described below. After pasteurization, if you're ready to use any plant parts right away, you can crush them for immediate use or store the larger parts in a container for preservation.

This technique is also ideal for harvesting seeds from flowers and harvesting flower parts. The seeds will fall out of the flower, so be sure to place your collection method close enough to the flower to ensure you can collect all the seeds.

Another method that's ideal if you have a big harvest for one plant and the climate is warm or hot is to place your plant parts on organic cotton, let them dry in the sun, and then make an indoor clothesline in a warm, dry, dark place. Use two ropes and clothespins to pull the sheet taut on both ends so that all the plant parts are in one uniform layer until they're dry.

Then, you can sort leaves, stems, and flowers and place each plant part in a thick paper bag or organic pillowcase so that you can crush the plant parts before pasteurizing and preserving them in a glass airtight container.

You can also do "vine drying" while they're still in containers or in the garden and the plant has been sun-dried. Remove the stems when the plant is completely dry and crispy to the touch.

For freshly plucked roots, chop the roots into smaller portions, place on a cookie sheet, and dry in the oven at 100°F.

Freezing Techniques

Freezing is a good method for extracting essential oils from herbs, for delicate herbs, and for mixing herbs into cooking recipes. Start by washing the plant and patting the parts with a clean cotton cloth until they're dry. Place the plant parts in glass containers with airtight lids and put them in the freezer. You could also freeze them on trays before they go into airtight containers. For food safety, the goal is to freeze the plants as rapidly and uniformly as possible to minimize ice crystal formation and freezer burn, which negatively affects the quality (NCHFP 2024).

Storage Preparation

There are many ideal storage techniques for all plant parts, starting with one necessary method to ensure safe storage: pasteurization.

The pasteurization process kills any insects and eggs that attach to plants. There are two techniques for pasteurization: freezing and heating (Herman 2021).

▸ With the freezing method, place the dry plant part in the freezer for at least 48 hours.

▶ With the heating method, place the plant in a single layer on a cookie sheet and cook in a preheated oven at 160°F for about thirty minutes. Transfer to a cooling rack until the plant parts are totally dry and not warm to the touch to prevent mold so that they can be safely stored in an airtight glass container (NCHFP n.d.).

Key Storage Tips

▶ Store your plant parts in large parts in glass airtight containers, ideally tinted glass, to minimize damage from light. Please avoid using plastic containers that could negatively impact the quality of your herbs.

▶ Your storage space should be cool, dark, and dry, with adequate ventilation.

▶ Make sure you label the harvesting and storage date for every container. The shelf life of properly preserved dried foods ranges from four months to one year depending on the plant part and the temperature of your storage space: at 60°F, your plant parts should be safe for one year, but at 80°F, the shelf life drops to six months.

▶ Once your plants are properly stored, check the glass jars periodically for signs of moisture. If there's any sign of spoilage, discard the contents. If there's no sign of spoilage, you can re-dry and repackage (NCHFP 2024). To ensure food safety, single-use containers are ideal if you plan on opening your containers often because every time you open a container of dried or frozen food, it gets exposed to air, moisture, and other potential contaminants.

▶ For frozen food, look out for ice crystal formation and freezer burn.

Pantry of Plenty

Now that you have a healthy stock of safe dried and frozen herbs, you're ready to start making organic herbal remedies and homemade products to green your home and nature. First, let's take some well-deserved time to learn about the herbal remedies that reduce anxiety and stress, boost mood, promote mental health, and help us heal from physical and emotional trauma. We'll also look at healing techniques that help us gain emotional balance, peace of mind, and a healthy mind–body connection.

"Knowledge is power. Sharing knowledge is the key to unlocking that power."

– MARTIN UZOCHUKWU UGWU

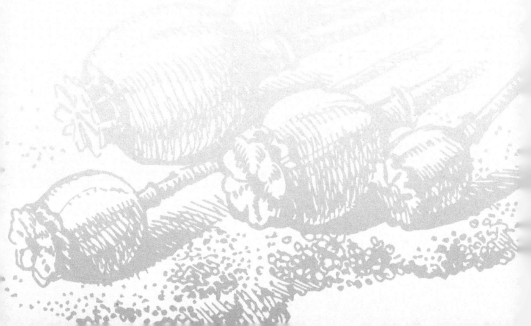

IN THE SPIRIT OF OUR ANCESTORS...

M y journey with herbal remedies began with a health scare, and I often wonder now if I'd have gotten so sick in the first place if I'd known what our ancestors knew about natural healing. Perhaps it was a health scare that brought you here too, or maybe it was concern about keeping your family healthy in the most natural way possible. Whatever the reason, there's always a trigger that sends people looking for natural solutions, and that's because we've become so far removed from the knowledge that used to be passed down between the generations. As a society, we rely heavily on pharmaceutical drugs, and while, of course, there's a place for these, they often address the symptoms rather than the cause, and we end up falling sick again.

We're blessed by living in modern times: We can combine both ancient wisdom and modern medicine to keep ourselves healthy... Yet it seems we've gone too far the other way, and we know little about the natural remedies that could be protecting our health. Having made such a difference in my own life by learning about herbal medicine, I've become determined to help more people connect with this ancient wisdom, aiming to share it just as our ancestors did. If you'd like to join me on this valuable mission, you can do so very easily: All you have to do is write a short review.

By leaving a review of this book on Amazon, you'll spread the information that our ancestors knew and help other people who are looking for it to find it.

There are many ways information can be shared, and a review is a powerful one: It helps people to find the information they're looking for and determine whether they've found the right resource for them. Our ancestors passed this knowledge on through word of mouth, but we have many more tools at our disposal now. I truly believe that if we use them, we can bring this important knowledge back into the collective consciousness.

Thank you so much for your support. Your words have more of an impact than you might realize.

"Healing is a matter of time, but it is sometimes also a matter of opportunity."

– HIPPOCRATES

CHAPTER SIX

Take Control of Your Mind, Body and Spirit

Herbal Remedies for Mental Health and Wellness

W e've all had a "gut feeling" about something in our lives. Maybe it's an intuitive feeling, or maybe it involves an emotional response to a situation or person. Whatever the reason, our emotions affect our bodies and vice versa. In this chapter, we'll explore the plant-based and herbal remedies that can boost our moods, calm our bodies and minds, heal trauma, feed our souls, and support our spiritual lives and rituals. Let's start in the gut.

The Gut Microbiome

Did you know that you have two brains? One is in your head, and the other one is in your gut, specifically your enteric nervous system (ENS), which has a two-way connection to the central nervous system. This means the gut and the brain are always talking via a complex network of nerve cells, microbes, and chemicals. This system includes the vagus nerve, which stretches from the brain all the way to the colon; the gut microbiome, where trillions of microorganisms live, and neurotransmitters that relay information between the brain; and the digestive tract. This system regulates everything from digestion to emotions and moods. Medical science has only recently started exploring this superhighway, discovering that the gut microbiome produces a whopping 95 percent of the body's total serotonin, which aids digestion and sleep and is an incredible antidepressant and mood-enhancer. The gut also produces GABA, known to reduce stress, anxiety, and fear (Appleton 2018). The gut is also talking to the immune system, which fights harmful viruses and bacteria in both the brain and the gut, where bacteria impact cytokines linked to the body and the brain's inflammatory responses (Cassano 2024).

There's probably good reason that we have sayings like "Follow your gut" and "gut feeling." Research has found that mental health issues like anxiety are linked with Irritable Bowel Syndrome, and clinical studies have linked depression and self-reported lower quality of life with fewer specific gut microbes. A low-quality diet of fast foods and processed foods causes inflammation and may also be linked to depression. That's why there's a new field called psychobiotics, focused on the potential benefits of probiotics on mental health. Clinical research has shown a potential link between probiotics and decreased social anxiety (Cassano 2024).

Our gut contains good gut bugs and bad gut bugs that need to feed off the foods we eat to survive. It's a sort of survival of the fittest world. If we feed good gut bugs, they'll multiply and diversify the microbiome. If we feed the bad gut bugs, they'll do the same.

Four Types of Microbiome–Healthy Foods

There are four types of foods that our good gut bugs prefer to eat. Scientific research has found that they're significantly linked to human health and disease treatments (Wang et al. 2024):

Probiotics are live bacteria found in fermented foods, including yogurt with active bacterial culture, kimchi, miso, kefir, sauerkraut, and some cheeses. Research has found that they may protect and heal the liver from damage and may treat psychiatric disorders and chronic hypertension.

Prebiotics are molecules that stimulate beneficial microbes, and they're found in many vegetables, including garlic, onions, leeks, asparagus, bananas, artichokes, and chicory root. They're also in legumes like lentils and chickpeas and in some mushrooms and whole grains like barley, rye, and oat.

Synbiotics are a combination of probiotics and prebiotics. You can make a delicious, gut-friendly meal or snack by mixing the above-mentioned ingredients.

Postbiotics are a sort of digestive tract for gut bugs in the form of waste material called metabolites. Scientists know that the gut microbiome produces hundreds of postbiotic chemicals linked to good health, including vitamin K, B Vitamins, antimicrobials, antibacterials, and anti-inflammatory fatty acids that protect the gut lining and help with metabolism. Clinical research has found that postbiotics can treat bacterial resistance from overuse of antibiotics that disrupt the gut's microbiota, and one study found that adding blackcurrant extract provided an extra boost (Wang et al. 2024).

Plants For Antibiotic Resistance

Overuse of antibiotics has made antimicrobial resistance (AMR) one of the most serious threats to human health; in Europe, it was linked to over 300,000 deaths in 2015, and it can't target specific pathogens, so it impacts the whole microbiome, eradicating all the good bugs. Researchers looked at gut microbiomes in twenty countries and found that healthy people not taking antibiotics had a five-fold abundance of antimicrobial resistance genes, and the countries with the highest abundance included Spain, France, and China, three countries with a high use of antibiotics. The lowest rates were found in countries that had lower rates of antibiotic usage, including the Netherlands and Germany (Lee et al. 2023). Antibiotics are designed to treat bacterial infections, but they're overused for minor infections and viral and fungal infections. Many plants and herbal remedies provide excellent antibacterial capabilities so that people can avoid overuse of antibiotics. Some of the best include garlic, ginger, echinacea, myrrh, thyme, goldenseal, oregano, and cloves (Pietrangelo 2024).

Herbal Prebiotic and Probiotic Remedies

Modern medical research into two Ayurveda herbal medicines connected to gastrointestinal health—licorice and slippery elm—found that they provided a significant positive increase of microbiota and that consumption, particularly of licorice, may lead to improved gut health and treat many digestive disorders (Peterson et al. 2018). Another study found that flaxseed and chicory root had prebiotic benefits and that licorice, curcumin, and herbs containing tannins and anthocyanins had potentially bioactive metabolites (Thuman et al. 2019).

Tannin-rich plants include yarrow, witch hazel, meadowsweet, horsetail, red raspberry, cocoa, chamomile, cinnamon, peppermint, rhubarb yerba mate, coffee, and of course, green and black teas. Keep in mind that soaking and cooking these plants can reduce the tannins.

Anthocyanin herbs are typically found in plants with pigments of red, blue, and purple, including many berries, particularly mulberries, black elderberries, and black currants.

Herbal Remedies for Mental Health and Wellness

Since ancient times, we've relied on plants to improve our mood, de-stress and calm our minds, get better sleep, heal emotional trauma, and engage in spiritual practices and rituals. Today, one in five Americans take psychiatric medications, a 22 percent increase since 2001 (Willson 2024). Yet research has shown that these medications may be ineffective and linked to debilitating side effects. A recent systematic review looked at 102 studies and found that for many mental illnesses, medications were only effective for 33 percent of people with depression, compared to 43 percent who used psychotherapy options, like talk therapy. Overall, the effect sizes of most medications to treat many psychiatric "disorders" were small or medium, with overall response rates of less than 50 percent. The researchers concluded that "after more than half a century of research, thousands of [clinical trials] and millions of invested funds, the 'trillion-dollar brain drain' associated with mental disorders is presently not sufficiently addressed by the available treatments (Leichsenring et al. 2022)." Meanwhile, medication side effects are common, and a systematic review found that for children and teens, the risk of suicide and aggression doubled (Sharma et al. 2016). Let's look at ideal plant and herbal remedies for each area of health and wellness, but please keep in mind that taking any herbal remedy, particularly a combination of psychiatric medications and herbal medicines, may cause significant adverse effects (Siwek, et al. 2023), so please consult with your doctor first.

Herbal Medicines for Stress

Ashwagandha

Ashwagandha is an Indian Sanskrit name that combines ashwa (horse) with gandha (smell), because this shrub smells like a wet horse. Also known as Indian ginseng and winter cherry, it's used in Ayurveda as an adaptogen, literally meaning that it helps people adapt and become more resilient to emotional and biological stressors. The Latin name for this shrub is *Withania somnifera* (the *somnifera* means sleep) and it's also used to reduce stress, anxiety, and cognitive issues. Ashwagandha is rich in phytonutrients, including alkaloids and steroidal lactones. Clinical studies have linked intake of the root, the root and the leaf, and dried root power with curbing anxiety, fatigue, and cortisol levels; beneficial dosages were in the 500-600mg/day range, but some studies using the root and dried root powder involved much higher dosages. Another study found that participants taking 225-400 mg/day of a root and leaf extract had less stress, anxiety, and depression and lower cortisol than the placebo group. Many other studies have found similar benefits, with common side effects like digestive issues, nausea, and drowsiness; some people had more serious liver injury, though researchers acknowledge that some products contained other ingredients, and these trials were done over three months, so it's unclear whether long-term use could cause serious side effects. It may interact with pharmaceutical treatments, including hormonal thyroid medications, and it's not recommended for pregnant women and men with prostate cancer (NIH 2023).

Catnip

Catnip isn't just for cats—it's good for us too! It belongs to the mint family, and its potency lies in the dried leaves and white flowers; the root is a stimulant. Leaves and flowers are typically used in teas to treat insomnia, anxiety, and headaches. For catnip tea, mix two teaspoons of dried leaves or flowers with a cup of boiled water and steep for up to fifteen minutes. Mixing with lemon brings out the minty taste. Keep in mind that it will cause drowsiness and is a diuretic, and avoid it if you're pregnant or have pelvic inflammatory disease, as it can cause uterine contractions (Gotter 2018).

Herbal Medicines for Depression and Anxiety

St. John s Wort

St. John's wort is a flowering shrub native to Europe that blooms on the birthday of John the Baptist, when people used to have a feast to celebrate and collect the bright yellow flowers. Today, in Europe, it's the most popular antidepressant, in part because it's been tested in a large number of clinical trials and linked to efficacy for mild to moderate depression; in some cases, it was found to be just as effective as tricyclic medications, which can cause many side effects (Mayo Clinic 2023). It may also be an effective alternative to pharmaceutical selective serotonin reuptake inhibitors (SSRIs) because it increases the availability of some neurotransmitters, including serotonin, dopamine, and norepinephrine (Brazier 2024). It's also effective at treating anxiety and menopause. The active parts are the leaves and flowers. It can negatively interact with many pharmaceuticals, including SSRIs, is not recommended during pregnancy and breastfeeding, and supplement use has been linked to anxiety, dizziness, diarrhea, fatigue, insomnia, and headache.

Valerian

Valerian was a favorite of Greeks and Romans and used to provide relaxation. It gets its name from the Latin word *vale*, which was used as a salutation that meant anything from "safe travels" to "sleep well"; it was used as a perfume, a body deodorant, and a diuretic. Hippocrates noted it as a gynecological and postpartum medicinal. It was also popular in the Middle East and in ancient India as incense for religious ceremonies (Touwaide and Appetiti 2023). The root is an anxiolytic that increases GABA levels in the brain, meaning it relieves anxiety, and some medical clinical studies have shown that taking the root extract may significantly reduce anxiety and reduce blood pressure and heart rate. It can cause drowsiness, headaches, nausea, vivid dreams, and nightmares, so please talk to your doctor about usage first, especially if you're already taking medications, including other herbal sedatives (Talkspace 2023).

Herbal Medicines for Emotional Trauma

Medical science has validated what the ancient herbal practitioners knew: that posttraumatic stress disorder can cause inflammation, oxidative stress, excessive free radicals in the brain, mitochondrial dysregulation, higher retention of aversive memories, and even neuron death (de Munter et al. 2021). At this point in the book, I hope you appreciate that so many herbal medicines can provide prevention and protection against many of these physiological issues. Let's look at a few more.

Hawthorn

Hawthorn has deep roots in ancient spiritual and healing practices. In various cultures, it's a symbol of love, good luck, protection, healing, alleviating emotional stress, and providing solace when you're grieving. It's sacred to American Indigenous people as a connection between the physical and spiritual worlds, a guardian of dreams, and a potent medicinal to treat the heart and digestion and cleanse the body, mind, and spirit. The Celtics viewed it as a link to the supernatural world of fairies and immortals, where you'd be cursed if you dared to cut down a hawthorn tree. In folklore, it's said to mend a broken heart and protect against evil spirits and malevolent forces. People would collect the leaves, twigs, berries, and thorns in a pouch or amulet and wear it or place it at their front door, and fortunetellers used sticks as divining rods. The Ancient Greeks and Romans associated it with love, romance, and fertility. Modern research has also linked it to heart health, so if you're not into rituals and talismans, you can always make tea with the leaves, flowers, and berries (Terry 2023). But please check for contraindications first.

Ginkgo Biloba

Ginkgo biloba has many benefits, which I mentioned in Chapter Two. It's also effective for PTSD. Clinical research found that earthquake survivors diagnosed with PTSD had significant benefits from taking ginkgo 200mg over twelve weeks (Wahbeh et al. 2015).

Herbal Medicines for Women

Dong Quai

Dong Quai is a traditional Chinese Medicine used for menstrual disorders, known as "female ginseng" and a "women's tonic." The root contains phytoestrogens that may regulate hormonal imbalances, irregular menstrual cycles, PMS, menopause symptoms, and pain and anemia. In TCM, it's ingested as a tea, tablet, or tincture. Dosages vary, so speak to a TCM practitioner and your doctor and avoid if you're pregnant, are taking any blood-thinners, or have any estrogen-sensitive diseases, including breast and ovarian cancer (Ames 2023).

Red Raspberry Leaf

Red raspberry leaf is used in Ayurveda as a "pita dosha" (meaning "to digest things"), to lower the body's heat and inflammation, and also balance and cool down emotions, including restlessness, anger, and self-criticism (Timmons 2020; Ajmera 2023). It contains calcium that helps strengthen bones, as well as magnesium, potassium, and Vitamin A. It may help with PMS symptoms and perimenopause and boost fertility by strengthening the uterus and helping it contract after labor. Many women drink it as a tea, using fresh or dried leaves, but it may cause diarrhea or nausea. Check with your doctor first, especially if you're pregnant, breastfeeding, or have any health disorders (Ajmera 2023).

Herbal Medicines for Men

Saw Palmetto

Saw palmetto is a palm tree with saw-like stalks. Indigenous Americans used the berries as an aphrodisiac and a sedative. It may improve prostate and urinary health, balance hormones, and enhance hair growth. Typically, the berries are eaten fresh or dried to make tea. There are a few reports of serious side effects, so talk to your doctor first (Petre 2023).

Horny Goat Weed

Horny goat weed is used in TCM as a tonic and aphrodisiac, and it's also known as "fairy wings," "Bishop's Hat" and "rowdy lamb herb." We know it has more than two hundred compounds and has become a popular herbal supplement to boost testosterone and curb erectile dysfunction.

Preclinical research has found it shares similar mechanisms to Viagra, and rat studies have shown some promise, but clinical research on people using the weed has yet to back up these claims (Guerrini 2023). As always, talk to your doctor first.

Traditional Spiritual and Ritual Plants

Whatever your spiritual or religious beliefs, the natural world is a great source of energy and solace, replenishing the mind and body and inspiring personal growth, creativity, inspiration, wisdom, well-being, and mindfulness, Our lives are interconnected with nature, and we rely on it for all aspects of life. Whenever I'm surrounded by nature, I feel my best. Whether I'm foraging for fresh medicinal plants (which we'll talk about in the next chapter), meditating on a beach, or tending my garden of plants, I'm mindful of the incredible fact that they take such great care of me. In return, I treat nature with respect, decency, gratitude, and reverence. I'm constantly reminded of our ancient ancestors who worshipped the natural world and believed that plants are intelligent, conscious, spiritual beings.

Many herbal practitioners focus exclusively on the spiritual powers of plants and think about physical and psychological illnesses as a side effect of spiritual and emotional imbalance. Many of them don't give much of a sod about the modern scientific evidence—they see herbalism through the lens of spirituality, not through a microscope. I like a good balance of these two ends of the spectrum, but let's focus on the mystical elements and the unexplainable mysteries of nature that people still lean on for rituals, ceremonies, and spiritual healing and growth. To me, this is a necessary step to the holistic approach.

Plants are highly responsive to their environment for survival. The air, the soil, the water, the local ecosystem, and the animals that live among them are integral. Plants, like everything else that exists today, adapt to challenges by developing a powerful immune system that can face challenges from weather changes to pests, including human pests that have increasingly encroached on and exploited nature. Plants have all sorts of traits that help them adapt to changes and harness the capabilities of other plants. In all parts of the globe, from China to India to South America, we have leaned on them as potent partners in spiritual rituals and ceremonies since ancient times.

Indigenous American healers and shamans use many herbs in rituals to support spiritual health, including aloe, dandelion, echinacea, goldenseal, sage, tobacco, and plant-based psychedelics. Across the pond, Traditional African medicinal healers have long cherished many herbs used for health and healing rituals, alongside prayers and dancing, including aloe, ginger, honeybush, and devil's claw. In Ayurveda, medicinal plants are part of a holistic approach to well-being, combining a balanced diet with physical exercise, meditation, and yoga that emphasizes breathwork, massage therapy, and rituals. Since ancient times, Iranian and Islamic practitioners have taken a similar holistic approach, calling it "mizaj," a term for temperament in people and everything else in nature. In Australia, prior to colonization, spiritual doctors had higher status than their "medicine men" assistants. These are just some examples of the many cultures of the world that rely on plants for spiritual and emotional health and for rituals and ceremonies, imbuing plants with the same essential qualities and rights as humans (Boye 2024).

Many plants have long been relied upon to promote spiritual health and ward off negative forces. Bay leaves and kava were said to stimulate prophetic dreams; angelica was said to exorcise demons; dandelion was a direct line to the spirit world; cinnamon stimulated psychic powers; and yarrow was used in meditation and for building psychic connections. Let's focus on two additional plants that hold unique allure in many cultures for their potency as spiritual and emotional guides.

Mugwort

Mugwort is sacred to many Indigenous cultures and has been used for centuries; called the "holy of holies" and the "mother" of all the revered healing herbs, in part because it's popular with women's fertility rituals and divination rituals around different stages of women's lives, including to sync the moon and menstrual cycles, both of which are twenty-eight-days. In fact, the modern name comes from the Greek *menus*, which means moon and power. This holy plant is believed to enhance psychic powers, allow us to communicate with ancestors, tap into our unconscious minds, cleanse our bodies and souls, and stimulate dreams (Martinez 2023). Medieval Europeans used it to ward off evil spirits, Chinese people still use it during dragon boat festivals to do the same, it's used in TCM as an alternative to tobacco, and it's burned during acupuncture.

Jasmine

Jasmine means "gift from God" in Persian. The white, star-shaped petals bloom at night, filling the darkness with its distinct sweet fragrance, revered by perfumiers, fortune tellers, and love potion spell-casters. It's a symbol of peace among Middle Eastern cultures, and Buddhists adorn their temples with the flowers, connecting them to motherhood, birth, and enlightenment. A dab of jasmine oil is said to stimulate serotonin and provide relief from stress, anxiety, depression, insomnia, and trauma; in aromatherapy, it's also a meditation aid, believed to help with mental clarity, focus, and mindfulness (Organica Botanicals 2023). The Chinese have made jasmine tea since the 1300s, and in TCM, it's still touted for its uplifting "yang" qualities. Recent medical research has found it contains antimicrobial, anti-inflammatory, and antioxidant compounds, including GABA, a mood-booster. You can make tea with the flowers or essential oils, mixed with green tea if you need energy, or other herbal teas. Use hot but not boiled water to preserve the antioxidants (Levy 2024). If you want to grow jasmine, it requires warm temperatures of 60-75°F, about six hours of direct sunlight, and well-draining soil, and if you live in a cold climate, bring it indoors during winter and repot every three years. Some species will bloom for up to two months, but in warm climates, they could bloom year-round (Gillette 2024).

An Alternative Path to Mental Wellness

Now that you have some options for organic plants and herbs that stimulate the brain-gut axis and provide beneficial mental, emotional, and spiritual health and wellness, you'll become much more self-empowered and possibly less reliant on medications. Now, we're going to turn to making herbal remedies of personal and home cleaning products that are great for us and our ecosystem.

"Herbs are the friend of the physician and the pride of the cooks."

— CHARLEMAGNE

CHAPTER SEVEN

Ignite Your Creativity

Homemade Herbal Remedies and DIY Home Cleaning Products

D id you know that even when a product's called or even labeled organic, it isn't totally sustainable and free of chemicals, pollution, and synthetic pesticides and herbicides? In the US, the Department of Agriculture is responsible for certifying all operators, and they also do annual inspections. There are three grades of organic labeling (USDA n.d.): 100 percent organic; organic (95 percent of the product is certified organic); and "made with" organic (70 percent organic ingredients). Organic produce must contain only natural fertilizers, no GMOs, and no artificial colors, flavors, and preservatives; these products are also "traced from farm to store" by experts in organic farming. Operators are not allowed to plant on land that wasn't previously designated organic for three years before harvesting an organic crop, and they're prohibited from using genetic engineering, ionizing radiation, and sewage sludge (USDA n.d.). Yet some synthetic substances are still allowed, which includes many products and chemicals that I don't want in my food and herbal medicines. You can check out the full list here: https://www.ams.usda.gov/rules-regulations/organic/national-list

The Organic Trade Association (OTA) states that the benefits of organic products include reduced public health risks for farm workers, their families, and consumers, particularly children who face higher risks from traditional industry pesticides. Organic foods have also been shown to have higher nutritional value, and they have many environmental benefits, from absorbing carbon dioxide in the air to restricting the use of chemical fertilizers that deplete soil and contaminate water. Research from Western European countries has also found that organic farms have 34 percent more plant, insect, and animal species than conventional farms (OTA n.d.), so biodiversity is an eco-friendly feature.

I prefer to support local organic farmers and avoid Big Food supermarkets, but when I meet an organic farmer at a local farmer's market, I ask a lot of questions about their practices and the types of fertilizers and natural pesticides they use. If possible, I highly recommend going directly to a farmer's facility to check out the farm and the surrounding area, just like the recommendations for foraging. Once your own sustainable garden bears fruits, vegetables, and herbs, you can trade products and knowledge with other local producers.

The OTA recently issued a report called "US Organic Hotspots and Their Benefits to Local Economies," featuring many counties that have a high number of organic farms, including Monterey County (California), Huron County (Michigan), Clayton County (Iowa) and Carroll County (Maryland). Check out the full list to see if your region is a hotspot: https://www.ota.com/hotspots

I think the best way to guarantee our herbal remedies and personal products are 100 percent organic and eco-friendly and made with the best ingredients is to grow and make them ourselves. In this chapter, I'll show you how to make herbal remedies straight from your garden, and then I'll talk about the DIY household and personal products that you can make—they're ideal for our health, and they're sustainable, and they're ideal for the planet.

A Step-by-Step Guide to Homemade Herbal Remedies

Now that your herbs are safely stored, I'll guide you through the process of making infusions, decoctions, infused oils, salves, creams, tinctures, and syrups. Before you start making any remedy, it's a good idea to check for potential allergies. Once you've done an allergy check, you should start using a small amount of these herbal remedies to assess any unwanted side effects and then increase the amounts gradually.

If you have your own recipes ready to go, a general rule of thumb with herbs is that one teaspoon of dried, powdered herbs is equivalent to one tablespoon of the fresh ingredient (Gaifyllia 2024).

Herbal Tea Infusions

If you love to drink tea (I'm obsessed with it), this is a nice method to make an infusion with herbal medicines, though some herbals aren't very flavorful or are downright bitter. For the hard-to-swallow herbs, you can add other tasty herbs like licorice root, cinnamon, and ginger, and flavor with organic honey or lemon. You can make tea with dried, frozen, or fresh herbs. By adding water to your herbs, you'll benefit from much of the plant part's medicinal potency, but it's not ideal for plant parts that are high in resins and alkaloids, in which case the ideal solvent is alcohol (Blankespoor 2023).

- Stainless steel tea filters are ideal for preparing single-use fresh or dried infusions.

- If you're using one teaspoon of dried herb or one tablespoon of fresh herbs the general rule of thumb is to use one cup of water or eight ounces.

▸ For larger batches with fresh herbs, the folk method is to use one handful of herbs and one quart of water. Though some herbs have much higher potency, so be sure to research the herb's level of potency.

▸ If you prefer to measure by weight, mix 5.5 grams of dried herb with one cup of water.

▸ To make larger batches, you can use a French press, a bamboo infuser, or a ceramic pot. Once the infusion cools, transfer it to mason jars and make sure you label them with the date.

▸ Generally, the daily dosage for herbal remedies is three cups per day, based on a person weighing about 150 pounds. I recommend starting with one cup per day for the first week to check for allergies and side effects and then increasing the dosage to two cups the following week (Talerico 2022).

▸ For children, you'll need to do more research to find out if the herb is recommended for use with children. The general rule is to divide the child's weight by 150 pounds. The same rule applies to tinctures based on the number of recommended drops per day.

Decoctions

Decoctions are simmered teas, the preferred method for consuming bark, roots, hard seeds, and mushrooms. Place the herb in water and bring it to a boil; place a lid on it and simmer for about twenty minutes. Strain and reserve the strained herbs because you can often repeat the process a few more times. Take note of the scent and the color of the first decoction, and if the next round has a similar smell and look, it still contains active ingredients. You'll need to store any leftovers in the fridge or freezer, in an airtight container.

Infused Oils

Infused oils can be used as edible oils for skin treatments. Infused oils are made by mixing the herb with an oil (ideally an organic, virgin, cold pressed oil) that's rich in fatty acids. For edible oils, choose olive, avocado, coconut, almond, hemp seed, or grapeseed oil; for topical oils, you might prefer jojoba or argan oil. Unless you plan on using the oil within a week or you're using a quick heat method to make your herbal oil, it's best to use dried herbs for infused oils because fresh herbs have moisture, which can cause the oil to mold and spoil. Infused oils stored in airtight containers can last up to a year (Chappell 2019).

There are two methods: quick heat method and cold infusion (Talerico 2022).

The cold infusion method takes more time, but it's ideal with delicate herbs.

1. Put the dried herbs into your airtight container until it's three-quarters filled.

2. Add the oil until the dried herbs are completely covered, or at a ratio of approximately one ounce of dried herb to five ounces of oil.

3. Seal, put a date label on, and store the jar in a dark place for at least two to three weeks and up to six weeks, if possible.

4. Once it's ready, place some cheesecloth inside a sieve or colander and let the oil strain into a clean bowl, ideally one with a pour spout. Let it drain for a while, then squeeze out any extra oil from the cheesecloth.

5. Transfer the oil into a new airtight container and store in a cool, dark spot. If you plan to use the oil regularly, use a few smaller jars so that you're not opening and closing your "master" jar all the time, exposing it to light, heat, and bacteria.

The quick heat method is a faster way to make infused oil.

1. For fresh herbs, chop them up into small pieces to increase the potency and place them in a slow cooker, crockpot, or double boiler.

2. Add oil until the herbs are covered and have an extra inch or two of water; it's approximately a 1:3 ratio of herb to oil for fresh herbs and 1:5 for dried herbs.

3. Gently simmer the mix at a temperature of approximately 110°F or a crockpot setting of "warm." Use a thermometer to adjust the heat. Don't put a lid on the pot (Chappell 2019).

4. Simmer for at least thirty minutes and up to five days for a more potent blend.

5. Let the mixture cool down before straining and storing, using the same method as above.

Salves

Salves combine infused oils with wax, such as beeswax or soy wax.

1. Put eight ounces of the infused oil in a double boiler.

2. Add one ounce of beeswax and stir until melted. If the mix is too soft, add more beeswax.

3. Place the mix in airtight containers while it's still warm and easy to pour.

4. Place the date on the mixture and store in a cool, dark spot; salves in properly sealed containers will last up to a year (Chappell 2019).

Creams

Creams are a combination of infused oils with wax and distilled water.

1. Start by combining three-quarters of a cup of infused oil with one ounce of wax and heat gently until the wax melts.

2. Let that mix cool, then transfer the mix to a blender or food processor and gradually add one cup of distilled water, blending at high speed as you add more water.

3. Store as described above.

Poultices and Compresses

Poultices and compresses are ideal if you need to apply herbal medicine to your skin to treat burns, cuts, bruises, or sore, painful joints and muscles.

1. Mix your crushed dry or chopped fresh herb with a paste made with water and a binding agent like flour, or use a thick binding agent like honey, glycerin, or oil.

2. You can apply the treatment directly to the skin or use a cloth, like muslin.

3. If you're using muslin, sandwich a two-inch layer of the herbal paste between two layers and apply the muslin to your skin for at least thirty minutes. You can refrigerate or freeze the muslin for future use.

Tinctures

A herbal tincture is a concentrated herbal remedy that requires alcohol or vinegar to extract the active components of a plant part. It's typically used for oral treatments and requires a glass dropper. Please educate yourself about the potential side effects of using this higher potency method and get your doctor's okay first (Fletcher 2023).

1. If you're using alcohol, it should be eighty to one hundred proof for fresh, water-soluble herbs or 180 proof for dried herbs.

2. Measure your dried or fresh herbs and place them in an airtight container.

3. Pour an equal amount of alcohol or vinegar into the container at a ratio of 1:1.

4. Store the container in a dark spot for at least six weeks; shake the container every few days to maintain the mixture.

5. Strain the plant parts from the liquid. If you plan to use the tincture often, use a few containers so that you're so that you're not opening and closing one container frequently, exposing it to light, heat, and bacteria. You can fill a small dropper with the tincture for immediate use. Herbal remedies typically require one or two drops of a tincture or one full sleeve.

6. Make sure you place a label with the date on all the containers.

Soaps

Soaps are quite easy to make. In the past, our ancestors used animal fat and wood ash, but nowadays, soaps are made with lye, also known as sodium hydroxide, which has strong alkaline qualities that can turn oils into soap. Here's a great recipe for soap (Berry 2018):

Equipment: lye and an airtight container for the lye; gloves and goggles to protect hands and eyes; another container for mixing soaps; a digital scale to measure ingredients by weight; a thermometer; a soap mold; some wood or stainless steel spatulas and spoons; and a hand blender. Don't use aluminum or non-stick pots or utensils because they react negatively to the lye. Be sure to handle the lye with care; when it's heated, there'll be strong fumes, so consider doing this prep work outside if possible, or use your stove's exhaust fan.

You will need 9.5 oz. distilled water or cooled herbal infusion; 3.85 oz. sodium hydroxide (lye); 12 oz. organic olive oil; 7 oz. organic coconut oil; 4 oz. organic shea butter or cocoa butter; 3.5 oz. organic sunflower or sweet almond oil; 1.5 oz. organic castor oil; and your preferred herbs, flowers, or organic essential oils.

Directions:

1. Put on your goggles and gloves.

2. Place the water or herbal infusion in a stainless steel or ceramic container.

3. Sprinkle the lye into the water and stir until the lye dissolves.

4. Place the container in a safe area, away from kids and pets, and allow the mix to cool for about forty-five minutes, until the temperature is approximately 100°F.

5. Next, melt the coconut oil and butter over low heat and gradually add the other oils. Cool until the oils are at 95°F.

6. Pour the cooled lye into the warm oils. Start stirring the mixture by hand and periodically use a hand blender to whip the mix, but

don't whip it too much, which will create air bubbles and cause the soap to thicken too rapidly.

7. Within about five to ten minutes, the mix will the consistency of pudding and leave a trace when you drizzle it. Pour the soap into molds and cover with wax paper. The soap should be set within two days.

8. Remove the soap from the molds, and if you're using a large mold, cut the soap into smaller bars.

9. Place the bars on wax paper or a cooling rack, cover with a cloth, and cure the bars for four to six weeks, periodically rotating the bars so that both sides cure evenly. If you see any cracks, remove the cloth and move the soap to a cooler spot.

Shampoo

It's quite easy to make a natural shampoo for hair, and you can also add dried herbs to the shampoo to provide medicinal benefits and fragrance. I'll start with the base ingredients and provide herbal options for specific hair types.

To make a basic shampoo, you will need half a cup distilled water or boiled water; one quarter cup of liquid castile soap (or use one of your own homemade soaps); two teaspoons of organic oil (jojoba, avocado, almond, or olive oil); and ten to twenty drops of essential oils

Put all of your ingredients in an airtight glass container and shake well before each use (Konie 2021).

If you want to customize your shampoo with therapeutic herb options, you can use homemade essential oils or dried herbs. (Be sure to check with a doctor first, especially for children, pregnant women, and people that take medications and have health conditions.) For dried herbs, boil the required half cup of water and add one tablespoon of dried herbs of your choice. Steep for at least four hours, strain with a cheesecloth, and add the other ingredients listed above (Judy n.d.).

- ▸ **For dry scalp/hair:** calendula, chamomile, elderflowers, lavender, marshmallow root, nettle, parsley leaf, and sage.

- ▸ **For oily scalp/hair:** bay leaf, lemon balm, lemon peel, lemongrass, peppermint, rosemary, and thyme.

- ▸ **For dandruff:** rosemary, eucalyptus.

- ▸ **For psoriasis:** turmeric, tea tree oil, and aloe vera gel can also be added to shampoos or placed directly on the scalp, but if using aloe vera, please read Chapter Three first for details on extracting the active parts from the toxic parts (Cirino 2024).

The Sustainable, All-Natural Home

Many cleaning products contain toxic chemicals, artificial colors, and artificial scents that are bad for us and for the environment. They can release hundreds of volatile organic compounds (VOCs) that are neurotoxic, cause an elevated risk of cancer, and harm the respiratory and reproduction systems. A recent medical study tested thirty products, including conventional cleaners, "green" cleaners, and fragrance-free "green" cleaners. Researchers identified 530 quantifiable VOCs, 193 considered hazardous, and 205 below quantifiable VOC limits. They found that conventional products had 2,458 ug/mg3 of VOCs, "green" products had 1036 ug/mg3, and fragrance-free "green" products had 373 ug/mg3 (Tempkin, et al. 2023). Another study found that more than one hundred common products had at least one but often multiple chemicals linked to cancer and reproductive and developmental issues. Some of these products emit VOCs for months after use, harming us and accounting for a whopping half of the VOCs that cause air pollution (Upham 2023).

It gets worse when these chemicals flow into the soil, natural water sources, and inadequate wastewater treatment facilities that send the disinfected water back to us. The water flowing out of our taps needs to be disinfected to fight dangerous water-borne diseases like cholera and typhus. But that disinfecting process produces hundreds of thousands of disinfection byproducts (DBPs) that are known to be hazardous to our health because they're cytotoxic, mutagenic, and carcinogenic. Yet most DBPs are unregulated, and they surpass permissible limits (Kalita 2024). According to the Environmental Working Group's Tap Water Database, for too many Americans, tap water "is like pouring a cocktail of chemicals," including "forever chemicals" (PFAS) like lead and arsenic, more than 160 unregulated contaminants, including industrial and agricultural contaminants linked to cancer, fertility problems, hormone disruption, and damage to the brain and nervous system, particularly in low-income communities. Government regulations have so far been ineffective; 324 contaminants have been detected in US regions that regulators consider legal, but they far exceed the research from scientific studies (EWG 2021).

These are the many reasons that I highly recommend home-made, organic products to disinfect your home and clean your clothes. There's a good chance you already have many of these great natural cleaning products in your cupboards. Ideal options include vinegar, baking soda, and lemons.

All-Purpose Cleaner

Mix equal parts water and vinegar in a glass bottle to clean the majority of surfaces, floors, glass surfaces, stovetops, toilet bowls, and bathroom tiles. It's a great way to disinfect and remove soap scum and hard water stains.

Vinegar is acidic, so do a spot test first on any natural stone surfaces, and don't use it on wood. You can also make use of used lemon wedges to clean many surfaces, including ceramic and porcelain.

Wood Furniture and Surface Cleaner

Mix one cup of olive oil with half a cup of lemon juice to make a natural wood polish. Lemons can also be used to clean brass and copper.

Drain Cleaner and De-Clogger

Mix one cup of heated vinegar with one cup of baking soda.

Oven Cleaner and Grease Remover

Make a paste of equal parts baking soda, lemon juice, and vinegar. Let the paste sit on surfaces for up to thirty minutes, scrub with some elbow grease, and use a wet cloth to remove the paste. It's also a great paste for washing pots and pans with baked-on grease, and for cleaning and deodorizing your washing machine.

Household Deodorizers

Baking soda is great at absorbing bad odors. You can put a bowl of it in your fridge and freezer, sprinkle it on carpets and upholstery, and place it in any spots with funky odors, including garbage cans and sneakers. It's also a great spot remover for acidic stains on clothing. If you want a spray option for your upholstery, carpets, and clothing, mix twenty-four ounces of hot water with one cup of baking soda until dissolved, place in a glass spray bottle, and add ten drops of essential oils to the mix.

Laundry Detergent

Here's the recipe for a good natural laundry detergent that's also low-sudsing (Leverette 2024): This recipe includes borax, baking soda, and sodium bicarbonate (washing soda). Baking soda and sodium bicarbonate are similar, but baking soda contains about half of the sodium of washing soda, which has a much higher pH, larger, courser crystals, and should never be consumed. Sodium bicarbonate can damage skin and eyes, so be sure to wear rubber gloves when you prepare this detergent. Sodium bicarbonate can also be harsh on clothing, so for a delicate fabric detergent (Corona 2023), try an alternative option provided below that's also borax-free. Borax is natural, but it can also cause lung, skin, and eye irritation, and should not be consumed (Hills 2022). Be sure to keep these two ingredients and the laundry detergent mix in sealed glass containers on a high shelf so that kids and pets can't reach them.

In a large, sealable container, mix one cup of pure soap flakes; one cup of baking soda; one cup of washing soda (sodium bicarbonate); and half a cup of borax (sodium borate).

1. Mix all the ingredients and seal the container.

2. You'll need about one half a cup of this laundry detergent per load in a top-load washer, or in a high-efficiency or front-load washer, two tablespoons per load.

3. If you're hand-washing the detergent, use about half a cup with four to five cups of water, and mix the water and detergent until dissolved before adding your clothing.

4. For mildewed items, like towels that still smell musty after washing, soak your items overnight with a combination of one cup of baking soda and two to four cups of water, enough to allow your items to be fully immersed.

5. Vinegar is a great natural fabric softener, so add one cup of vinegar prior to the rinse cycle. Keep in mind that baking soda and vinegar

will neutralize each other, so don't start a wash cycle by combining both.

6. If you need a borax-free and sodium bicarbonate-free alternative for babies or delicate garments, substitute borax and sodium bicarbonate with baking soda. If you're hand-washing clothing, soak the mixture for a half hour, stirring clothing periodically; rinse thoroughly, mix equal parts vinegar and water, soak for fifteen minutes, and rinse thoroughly.

7. A great natural fragrance-enhancer can be added to your laundry detergent by adding a few drops of essential oil with your laundry detergent prior to washing.

Homemade, Sustainable and Eco-friendly Herbs and Plants

Before I started making herbal remedies and household products, my priority was survival. But once my pantry was stocked with organic herbal remedies and homemade personal products that were good for me and the planet, I felt much more empowered, self-sufficient, and rooted in the natural world. I felt like I could finally thrive, no matter what happened in the future, and I felt more hopeful that the future could be brighter. I wanted to take my skills and knowledge to the next level. The only missing ingredient was a strong connection to my community and to other like-minded people in my neighborhood and around the world. So, let's get into that topic now so that we can make our world much greener, healthier, and more sustainable.

"If you think in terms of a year, plant a seed; if in terms of ten years, plant trees; if in terms of one hundred years, teach the people."

— CONFUCIUS

CHAPTER EIGHT

Cultivating Sustainability

Environmental Best Practices

S ustainability was always a foundational principle among our ancient ancestors. Today, the rising population and increased demand for both pharmaceuticals and medicinal plants and herbs have led to overharvesting, unmonitored cultivation and production, and for-profit exploitation of the natural world and the people who have helped these remedies survive for tens of thousands of years. According to research on more than five thousand medicinal plants, 13 percent are now threatened. Some countries and regions have established policies and strategies to curb overharvesting, including limiting the number of people that can harvest plants, gathering only the plant part with medicinal benefits, better seed dispersal options, and home gardening. Yet, regulations can restrict use by traditional medicine providers, limiting their ability to continue their ancient practices (Mateo-Martin et al. 2023).

The threat of extreme shortages and extinction is one of many reasons I think about plants in the same way that I think about humans and other animals. If we regard plants as integral to our natural world instead of as resources we can overharvest, we'll take the necessary steps to ensure their continued survival and growth. We should treat them with the same respect and appreciation that we have towards all of the earth's natural resources to sustain and maintain the balance of our ecosystem.

I hope that you're already practicing sustainability in your home garden and are starting to appreciate the benefits of herbal remedies. Please keep in mind that by becoming self-sufficient, we'll stop relying on store-bought herbal medicines that may be much less effective and even toxic to us—and to the planet's increasingly strained ecosystem. We're healing ourselves *and* the natural world. If you don't have the time, the resources, or the space to grow your own garden, or if you want to supplement your garden, this chapter will feature ethical, wildcrafting, and foraging techniques, tips for shopping at local farmer's markets, and community resources to help you connect with like-minded people and support a healthy, eco-friendly, self-sufficient community.

Let's start with the importance of biodiversity—the spice and the engine of a healthy ecosystem.

Biodiversity: The Key to Life

Diversity can be a good thing, and it's not just an overused buzzword for inclusivity. Biodiversity literally powers the world, ensuring the survival and health of everything on this incredible planet. But biodiversity requires balance and the cooperation of all plant and animal species on earth. We're the outliers in that mix. As I've already mentioned, our mass industrialization of agriculture and our overreliance on dirty energy and many other toxic pollutants have left the natural world teetering on the edge of destruction. In a biodiverse world, species evolve, and up to 98 percent ultimately become extinct. But scientists now estimate that the speed towards extinction has accelerated up to one thousand times, and many are warning that we're currently in the midst of the sixth mass extinction. Between 2001 and 2021, we lost 487 million hectares of tree cover, including 16 percent of mature forests and 1.9 million square kilometers of natural habitats. 28 percent of approximately 150,000 assessed species are now on the extinction level list, including one million animals and plants. We have lost 34 percent of conifers and 69 percent of cycads (Stallard 2023), ancient plants with stout and woody-trunked trees that typically live in tropical and subtropical climates, grow very slowly, and live a long time. But habitat destruction, climate change, and their popularity as ornamental plants have put this close relative of the ginkgo under threat (Mahr n.d.).

Keep in mind that 150,000 species is a drop in the earth's bucket of plenty. Scientists estimate that the true number of the earth's species is in the billions, or perhaps up to a trillion, if we include insects, fungi, bacteria, and single-cell organisms (Ritchie 2022). Let's also remember that many commercial herbal remedies on the shelves are not grown, harvested, and transported sustainably, and they often include toxic fillers and chemicals and low-quality mixtures of plant parts. By growing our own plants ethically and sustainably, we're consuming high-quality products that are ideal for the planet and us.

Biodiversity Tips for Your Garden

There are many ways to add biodiversity to a home garden. It'll benefit your garden, you, and the planet (Reynandez n.d.).

▶ **Plant at least some native and pollinator-friendly plants** to attract native species. Check out this site to find out more about your region's native plants and butterflies: http://nativeplant-finder.nwf.org/

▶ **Don't use chemical pesticides, herbicides, and fertilizers.**

▸ **Feed the birds.** They eat insects, pollinate plants, consume seeds, disperse them in droppings, and provide nutrients after they die. You can buy or make a birdhouse, a bird bath, and a bird feeder; keep the feeder stocked with seeds, like black-oil sunflower seeds. Be sure to clean the house, bath, and feeder often to prevent diseases. To find out more about the birds in your region, go to the interactive map at http://feederwatch.org/learn/common-feeder-birds/

▸ **Build houses for bats, butterflies, and bees.** Do your research for each species, and make sure that all the parts in these houses can be removed and cleaned every few months to prevent parasites and diseases.

▸ **Build a rain garden**, also known as a bioswale garden, to collect rainwater from your lawn, sidewalks, and roads. Rain gardens make use of water that puddles on surfaces to help remove pollutants from rainwater that ultimately ends up in local streams, rivers, and lakes; it will also attract all sorts of species—insects, butterflies, birds, and wild critters. For building tips, go to http://extension.umn.edu/landscape-design/rain-gardens

Ethical Foraging

Foraging for wild plants is a great way to learn to identify and differentiate specific plants and develop your survival skills. Ethical, sustainable foragers follow specific guidelines to ensure that they do it safely and respectfully:

▸ **Know the ecosystem.** Learn about the quality of the air, water, and soil to ensure that there are no industry pollutants and car pollution nearby.

▸ **Know your target plants and their look-alikes.** Before you start foraging in a specific region, educate yourself about the plants that grow in the region, including plants that look very similar to each other but may be poisonous. Brush up your identification skills in advance by reading local blogs and books about the region's wild plants. Connect with a local herbalist, wild forager, or other expert who offers an introductory class in that region's wild plants. There are also identification apps available, like PlantSnap. Another great resource is Eat the Planet, which has a lot of advice and tips for safe foraging and identification (Sweet n.d.).

▸ **Check the plant's conservation status** and learn about the plant's reproductive patterns to ensure you're harvesting a sustainable plant, including invasive species.

▸ **Know the picking rules.** National and regional parks often have no picking rules. Get permission first if you want to forage on private land.

▸ **Take safety precautions.** Bring a friend or tell another trusted friend where you're going and what time you'll be back. Pack a first aid kit in case you injure yourself while foraging, and if the region has bears, bring bear spray.

▸ **Check the weather** for potential storms and wildfire warnings.

▸ **Be prepared.** Pack thick gloves, a clean pocket knife, a few different containers to keep separate plants divided, a hat, sunscreen, and some food and water.

▸ **Take only what you need.** Once you identify an ideal plant, take only the plant parts you need. If you're targeting the root, you'll need to remove the entire plant, but if you only need the leaves, berries, flowers, and seeds, take only the part that you need. The appropriate quantity is typically no more than one-quarter of the plants or plant parts and be sure to leave the largest "mother" plants in place.

▶ **Target invasive species.** They're an exception to the one-quarter rule. Pick as much as you like.

▶ **Leave the area as you found it.** When you pick a plant, fill in any holes; be sure to leave the area like you found it or in better shape by picking up any trash that other people have left behind.

▶ **Take a sample.** If you're in any doubt about the identity of a plant, take only a small sample of that plant so that you can do follow-up research later to ensure the plant isn't toxic or overharvested.

▶ **Know the ideal methods for cooking and storing** that specific plant. You'll want to pasteurize all wild plants to get rid of insects and eggs.

Forging Strong Community Networks

Communities are the bedrock of human existence. We're social creatures, and our individual success, well-being, and survival are dependent on communication, support, and collaboration with others. There are so many ways to build lasting connections in your community and among herbal medicine practitioners in other parts of your country and the world. Here are some great options:

▶ **Eat local foods** produced close to home, ideally within a hundred miles of your location. *The 100-Mile Diet* is a book by two Canadian writers who consumed only local food for a year, providing an intimate journal of the benefits and challenges of eating local foods and avoiding the Big Food trap.

▶ **Start or join a community garden**, which can transform unused urban and suburban spots into productive gardens. Schools and community centers are also great sources for community projects, inspiring kids and all citizens to grow their own food and become eco-friendly.

▶ **Host a neighborhood compost pile** to green your street and neighborhood.

▶ **Start or join a local community-supported agriculture** program (CSA) to find local organic farmers; often, they'll deliver food straight to your door or have open-house days so that locals can tour their farms.

▶ **Attend local and regional conferences and workshops.** HerbRally is an excellent resource run by an Oregon duo. They provide podcasts, blog posts, a comprehensive list of herbal medicine schools, and an events calendar with regional and international conferences, workshops, fairs, festivals, apprenticeship opportunities, and even herb walks, searchable by state.
Other useful site for herb courses is https://bestonlineonline-herbalismcourses.com, which has a list of options, including https://commonwealthherbs.com.

▶ **Start or join a zero-waste program** in your community. Many states and regions certify zero waste facilities. In 2016, Mountain Rose Herb, an Oregon-based company that makes organic herbal remedies and provides bulk herbs, was the first company to receive platinum status for their close-to-zero waste policies; 96.2 percent of their waste was recycled and didn't end up in a landfill (Heidi 2020).

▸ **Connect with expert herbal medicine practitioners**, academics and businesses, including the American Botanical Council and its Sustainable Herbs Program, which provides sustainability and ethnobotany webinars.

▸ **Participate in forums**, such as Herbforum.org and Davesgarden.com, which has many farm and garden sections for many US states and other countries, including Australia and New Zealand.

▸ **Stay up-to-date on global and regional topics in traditional medicine** at the World Health Organization's hub for Traditional, Complementary and Integrative Medicine (https://www.who.int/health-topics/traditional-complementary-and-integrative-medicine). WHO also has a hub for Global Traditional Medicine Centre (http://www.who.int/initiatives/who-global-traditional-medicine-centre), which was launched in 2022 "as a knowledge hub, with a mission to catalyze ancient wisdom and modern science for the health and well-being of people and the planet (World Health Organization 2023)."

Together We Can Catalyze Positive Change

I hope that this book will help catalyze your journey to finding the light that our ancient ancestors provided, whether you're in the midst of a health and wellness crisis or you're trying to optimize your health with preventative options that might help you avoid a future health problem. When I faced my own health challenges, I realized that I had spent so much of my early life looking to the future or regretting things from my recent past that I couldn't possibly rewrite. Sure, it would have been ideal if I could have avoided the pain and suffering, but because those cracks appeared, I ultimately got to see the light shining through. That light reconnected me to my ancient ancestors and the natural world at a time in my life—and all our lives—when I needed it most. We've become too reliant on Big Food, Big Pharma, and other industries that pose serious threats to our health and well-being and that of our planet, which needs our help more than ever before. As individuals, we can do so much to help the planet and all its incredible species of plants and animals that nourish and sustain us. But our collective hope, energy, and actions will ultimately change the world for the better.

Now is the time to start giving back to the natural world. By following my eight steps of self-empowerment, you'll develop a holistic approach to life that will help you start implementing change in your life, your home, your community, and the world. I guarantee that if you take these steps with an open mind and a heartfelt desire to effect change, it will open the door to a world of possibilities. Many other people share your hopes and dreams of finding a better way to live—one that provides balance, stability, inspiration, wisdom, environmental sustainability, and both personal and collective health, wellness, and empowerment. I wish you the best of luck on this incredible journey. Together, we can carve a different path that's healthier for us and the natural world.

IN PURSUIT OF A HEALTHIER WORLD

We all share this planet, and taking care of our health in a natural way is good for us all. Take a moment now to share this knowledge and help other people to begin a transformative journey with herbal medicine.

By sharing your honest opinion of this book and a little about your own experience with using herbs for health, you'll spread the word and direct new readers to all the guidance they need to get started.

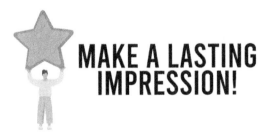

MAKE A LASTING IMPRESSION!

Thank you so much for your support. The wider we can spread this information, the healthier we'll all be—including the planet.

Check out these *OTHER* Endure Elite originals

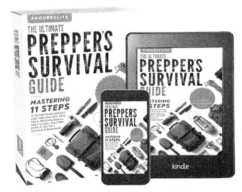

The *Ultimate* Prepper's Survival Guide

Or go to tinyurl.com/**PreppersGuide**

MORE ORIGINALS
COMING SOON

REFERENCES

15 Impactful knowledge-sharing quotes for your team! (2023, August 21). Bit Blog. https://blog.bit.ai/knowledge-sharing-quotes/

Aboelsoud, N. H. 2021. "Herbal Medicine in Ancient Egypt," Brewminate. June 22, 20 2021. https://brewminate.com/herbal-medicine-in-ancient-egypt/.

Ahn E. and Hyun Kang. 2018. "Introduction to Systematic Review and Meta-Analysis." Korean Journal of Anesthesiology 71 (2): 103-112. doi: 10.4097/kjae.2018.71.2.103. https://www.ncbi.nlm.nih.gov/pmc/articles/PMC5903119/.

Ajmera, R. 2023. "4 Benefits Of Raspberry Leaf Tea, From Experts In Ayurveda & Hormone Health." MGB Health. May 16, 20 2023. https://www.mindbodygreen.com/articles/raspberry-leaf-tea-benefits.

Alex, Bridget. 2019. "Prehistoric Medicine: How Archaic Humans Cured Themselves," Discover Magazine. May 10, 2019. https://www.discovermagazine.com/planet-earth/prehistoric-medicine-how-archaic-humans-cured-themselves.

Almanac. 2024a. "What are the 2024 Frost Dates?" The Old Farmer's Almanac. 2024. https://www.almanac.com/gardening/frostdates.

Almanac. 2024b. "2024 Planting Calendar." The Old Farmer's Almanac. 2024. https://www.almanac.com/gardening/planting-calendar.

Ames, Hana. 2023. "What Is Dong Quai and What Are Its Uses?" Medical News Today. November 8, 2023. https://www.medicalnewstoday.com/articles/dong-quai.

Appleton Jeremy. 2018. "The Gut-Brain Axis: Influence of Microbiota on Mood and Mental Health," Integrated Medicine (Encinitas) 17 (4): 28-32. PMID: 31043907.

Atkins. 2023. "Butterbur for Allergy Relief: Benefits and Uses." Expert Sinus Care. November 2, 2023. https://www.atkinssinus.com/butterbur-for-allergy-relief-benefits-and-uses/.

Barnes, A. 2022. "7 Research-backed Benefits of Cardamom and How to Use this Versatile Spice More Often." Business Insider. July 14, 2022. https://www.businessinsider.com/guides/health/diet-nutrition/cardamom-benefits.

Barry, Jan. 2018. "How to Make Your Own Soaps with Herbs." Mountain Rose Herbs. March 18, 2018. https://blog.mountainroseherbs.com/how-to-make-herbal-soap.

Blankespoor, Juliet. 2023. "Herbal Infusions and Decoctions: Preparing Medicinal Teas." Chestnut School of Herbal Medicine. June 9, 2023. https://chestnutherbs.com/herbal-infusions-and-decoctions-preparing-medicinal-teas/.

Bloom Institute. 2019. "How to Choose High Quality Herbs and Herbal Remedies." The Bloom Institute. September. 4, 2019. https://bloominstitute.ca/how-to-choose-high-quality-herbs/.

Boyle, Margaret. 2023. "Storing Garden Herbs for Cooking." The Old Farmer's Almanac. November 29, 2023. https://www.almanac.com/preserving-herbs.

Braverman, Jody. 2024. "Fennel: Health Benefits, Nutrients and Recipes." WebMD. April 16, 2024. https://www.webmd.com/food-recipes/health-benefits-fennel.

Bray, Freddy, Mathieu Laversanne, Hyuna Sung, Jacques Ferlay, Rebecca L. Siegel, Isabella Soerjomataram, Ahmedin Jemal. 2024. "Global Cancer Statistics 2022: GLOBOCAN Estimates of Incidence and Mortality Worldwide for 36 Cancers in 185 Countries." CA Cancer Journal for Clinicians 74 (3): 229-263. doi: 10.3322/caac.21834.

Brazier, Yvette. 2024. "St. John''s Wort: Should I Use it?" Medical News Today. January 12, 2024. https://www.medicalnewstoday.com/articles/174928.

Camilleri, Emma and Renald Blundell. 2024. "A Comprehensive Review of the Phytochemicals, Health Benefits, Pharmacological Safety and

Medicinal Prospects of *Moringaoleifera*." Heliyon 10 (6) doi: 10.1016/j.heliyon.2024.e27807.

Cassano, Olivia. 2024. "What is Your Gut-Brain Connection and What Role Does Nutrition Play?" Zoe.com. April 18, 2024. https://zoe.com/learn/gut-brain-connection.

Chappell, Sarah. 2019. "A Beginner"s Guide to Making Herbal Salves and Lotions." Healthline. December 18, 2019. https://www.healthline.com/health/diy-herbal-salves.

Chelu Mariana, Adina Magdalena Musuc, Monica Popa, Jose Calderon Moreno. 2023. "Aloe Vera-Based Hydrogels for Wound Healing: Properties and Therapeutic Effects." Gels 9 (7):539. doi: 10.3390/gels9070539.

Chen, David. 2023. "Will Thyme Oil Kill a Tooth Nerve?" Jackson Avenue Dental. December 16, 2023. https://www.jacksonavedental.com/post/will-thyme-oil-kill-a-tooth-nerve.

Chung, Emily. 2023. "How Supermarket Freezers Are Heating the Planet, and How They Could Change." CBC. January 29, 2023. https://www.cbc.ca/news/science/hfc-climate-supermarkets-1.6726627

Cirino, Erica. 2024. "Treating Scalp Psoriasis at Home, Naturally." Healthline. April 25, 24. https://healthlinerevive.com/health/scalp-psoriasis-home-remedies.

Colgate. 2024. "Garlic and Tooth Pain." Global Scientific Communications. February 12, 2024. https://www.colgate.com/en-ph/oral-health/brushing-and-flossing/how-to-use-garlic-to-cure-toothache.

Corona, Leslie. 2023. "Washing Soda and Baking Soda: What"s the Difference and Which is Better For Laundry?" Real Simple. December 29, 2023. https://www.realsimple.com/washing-soda-vs-baking-soda-8418441

Cowell, Whitney, Thomas Ireland, Donna Vorhees, Wendy Heiger-Bernays. 2017. "Ground Turmeric as a Source of Lead Exposure in the United States." Public Health Report 132 (3): 289-293. doi: 10.1177/0033354917700109.

Cronkleton, Emily. 2018. "How to Use Fresh Aloe Vera." Healthline. December 12, 2018. https://www.healthline.com/health/how-to-use-aloe-vera-plant.

Davison, Tamara. 2024. "The Environmental Impact of the Food Industry. CleanHub. March 14, 2024. https://blog.cleanhub.com/food-industry-environmental-impact.

de Munter, Johannes, Dimitrii Pavlov, Anna Gorlova, Michael Sicker, Andrey Proshin, Allan V. Kalueff, Andrey Svistunov, Daniel Kiselev, Andrey Nedorubov, Sergey Morozov, Alexsei Umriukhin, Klaus-Peter Lesch, Tatyana Strekalova, Careen A. Schroeter. 2021. "Increased Oxidative Stress in the Prefrontal Cortex as a Shared Feature of Depressive- and PTSD-Like Syndromes: Effects of a Standardized Herbal Antioxidant." Frontiers in Nutrition 8: 661455 doi: 10.3389/fnut.2021.661455.

Deering, Shelby. 2019. "Nature"s 9 Most Powerful Medicinal Plants and the Science Behind Them." Healthline. February 28, 2019. https://www.healthline.com/health/most-powerful-medicinal-plants.

Dehelean, Cristina, Iasmina Marcovici, Codruta Soica, Marius Mioc, Dorina Coricovac, Stela Lurciuc, Octavian Marius Cretu, Iulia Pinzaru. 2021. "Plant-Derived Anticancer Compounds as New Perspectives in Drug Discovery and Alternative Therapy." Molecules 19 (26): 1109. doi: 10.3390/molecules26041109.

Downey, Michael. 2023. "Spearmint Tea Quickly Boosts Mental Focus." Life Extension. August, 2023. https://www.lifeextension.com/magazine/2018/8/spearmint-tea-boosts-mental-focus.

Durant, Owen. 2014. "A World of Similarity: The Doctrine of Signatures and Its Application in Medicinal Plant Identification." Conference Paper, Herbal History Research Network, Royal Botanic Gardens Kew. June 2014. https://www.researchgate.net/publication/269688037_A_World_of_Similarity_The_Doctrine_of_Signatures_and_its_application_in_medicinal_plant_identification.

Eldridge, Lynn. 2023. "Adverse Reactions to a Medication or Drug." Verywell Health. May 24, 2023. https://www.verywellhealth.com/what-is-an-adverse-reaction-3959900.

EPA. 2024. "Composting at Home." United States Environmental Protection Agency. https://www.epa.gov/recycle/composting-home.

EPA. 2023. "Quantifying Methane Emissions from Landfilled Food Waste," Environmental Protection Agency, October, 2023. https://www.epa.gov/system/files/documents/2023-10/food-waste-landfill-methane-10-8-23-final_508-compliant.pdf.

EPA. 2022. "Sources of Greenhouse Gas Emissions." Environmental Protection Agency. 2022. https://www.epa.gov/ghgemissions/sources-greenhouse-gas-emissions#agriculture.

Everyday Roots. 2013. "Homemade Hot Pepper Cream for Arthritis & Joint Pain." Everydayroots.com. 2013. https://www.khromaherbs.com/blogs/news/cayenne-pepper-for-arthritis.

EWG. 2021. "State of American Drinking Water." Environmental Working Group. November, 2021. https://www.ewg.org/tapwater/state-of-american-drinking-water.php.

FAO. 2023. "Breaking the Plastic Cycle in Agriculture, Food and Agriculture Organization of the United Nations." May 6, 2023. https://www.fao.org/newsroom/story/Breaking-the-plastic-cycle-in-agriculture/en.

FDA. 2018. "The Drug Development Process." US Food and Drug Administration. January 4, 2018. https://www.fda.gov/patients/drug-development-process/step-3-clinical-research.

Firenzuoli Fabio and Luigi Gori. 2007. "Herbal Medicine Today: Clinical and Research Issues." Evidence Based Complement Alternative Medicine 4 (1): 37-40. doi: 10.1093/ecam/nem096. PMID: 18227931.

Fletcher, Jenna. 2023. "What is an Herbal Tincture? Recipes and Uses." Medical News Today. November, 22, 2023. https://www.medicalnewstoday.com/articles/324149.

Gaifillya, Nancy. 2024. "How to Convert Fresh to Dried Herbs Measurements." The Spruce Eats. March 3, 2024. https://www.thespruceeats.com/convert-herb-measurements-1706231.

Gillette, Barbara. 2024. "How to Grow and Care for Jasmine." The Spruce. June 6, 2024. https://www.thespruce.com/jasmine-growing-guide-8410140.

Goldman, Rena. 2017. "What is Comfrey?" Healthline. July 26, 2017. https://www.healthline.com/health/what-is-comfrey.

Gotter, Ana. 2018. "Catnip Tea." Healthline. September 18, 2018. https://www.healthline.com/health/catnip-tea.

Groves, Maria Noël. 2019. "Grow Your Own Herbal Remedies: How to Create a Customized Herb Garden to Support Your Health & Well-Being. Hachette Book Group.

Groves, Melissa. 2023. "12 Science-Backed Benefits of Peppermint Tea and Extracts." Healthline. March 10, 2023 https://www.healthline.com/nutrition/mint-benefits#TOC_TITLE_HDR_2.

Gu, Yaxin, Yimeng Wang, Keyun Zhu, Weihua Li, Guixia Liu, Yun Tang. 2024. "DBPP-Predictor: A Novel Strategy for Prediction of Chemical Drug-Likeness Based on Property Profiles." Journal of Cheminformatics 16 (4) doi: 10.1186/s13321-024-00800-9.

Guerrini, Giulia. 2023. "Horny Goat Weed." Examine. October 5, 2023. https://examine.com/supplements/horny-goat-weed/.

Gunnars, Kris. 2023. "10 Health Benefits of Turmeric and Curcumin." Healthline. November 27. 2023. https://www.healthline.com/nutrition/top-10-evidence-based-health-benefits-of-turmeric.

Hadjipateras, Elara. 2023. "Matcha Green Tea for Headaches & Migraines." Matcha.com. November 17, 2023. https://matcha.com/en-ca/blogs/news/matcha-green-tea-for-headaches-migraines.

Hassen, Gashaw, Gizeshwork Belete, Keila G. Carrera, Rosemary O. Iriowen, Haimanot Araya, Tadesse Alemu, Nebiyou Solomon, Diwas S. Bam,

Sophia M. Nicola, Michael E. Araya, Tadesse Debele, Michlene Zouetr, Nidhi Jain. 2022. "Clinical Implications of Herbal Supplements in Conventional Medical Practice: A US Perspective." Cureus 14 (7) doi: 10.7759/cureus.26893.

Heidi. 2020. "Mountain Rose Herbs: A TRUE Zero Waste Company." Mountain Rose Herbs. July 14, 2020. https://blog.mountainroseherbs.com/true-zero-waste-facility-certification.

Herbal Academy. n.d. "Herbal History: Roots of Western Herbalism." https://theherbalacademy.com/herbal-history/.

Herbal Academy. n.d. "How to Become an Herbalist: Understanding Herbal Certification." The Herbal Academy. ttps://theherbalacademy.com/understanding-herbal-certification/.

Herbaugh, Tracee. 2021. "Borage Seed Oil for Rheumatoid Arthrtitis." Medical News Today. September 6, 2021. https://www.medicalnewstoday.com/articles/borage-seed-oil-rheumatoid-arthritis.

Herman, Marilyn and Suzanne Driessen. 2021. "Preserving Herbs by Freezing or Drying." University of Minnesota, Food Safety Extension.

Hill, Ansly. 2022. "12 Benefits of Ginkgo Biloba (Plus Side Effects & Dosage)." Healthline. December 14, 2022. https://www.healthline.com/nutrition/ginkgo-biloba-benefits.

Hills, Jenny. 2022. "What is Borax and is it Safe to Use? The Real Facts About Borax and Its Many Uses." Healthy and Natural World. June 17, 2022. https://www.healthyandnaturalworld.com/borax/.

Hodge, Sharon. 2023. "Starting Seeds in Egg Cartons: Steps from Seed to Transplant." Utopia. March 30, 2023 https://utopia.org/guide/starting-seeds-in-egg-cartons-steps-from-seed-to-transplant/.

IQVIA. 2024. "The Global Use of Medicines 2024." IQVIA. January, 2024. https://www.iqvia.com/insights/the-iqvia-institute/reports-and-publications/reports/the-global-use-of-medicines-2024-outlook-to-2028.

Jerez Torres. 2022. "Homemade Plant Food: Tips for Helping Wilted Plants." Utopia. January 5, 2022. https://utopia.org/guide/homemade-plant-food-tips-for-helping-wilted-plants/.

Judy. n.d. "Homemade Herbal Shampoo." Green Valley Marketplace. https://www.greenvalleymarketplace.com/eat-right-live-well/judys-healthy-tips/homemade-herbal-shampoo/.

Kalita, Indrajit, Andreas Kamilaris, Paul Havinga, Igor Reva. "Assessing the Health Impact of Disinfection Byproducts in Drinking Water." ACS Publications 4 (4): 1564–1578. https://pubs.acs.org/doi/10.1021/acsestwater.3c00664?.

Khroma. 2017. "Benefits of Cayenne Pepper for Arthritis." Khroma Herbal Products, September 28, 2017. https://www.khromaherbs.com/blogs/news/cayenne-pepper-for-arthritis.

Konie, Robin. 2021. "All Natural DIY Shampoo." Thank Your Body. February 2, 2021. https://www.thankyourbody.com/all-natural-shampoo/.

Kumari, Binita. 2022. "Cardamom Cultivation: How to Grow The Queen of Spices, A Complete Guide!" Krishi Jagran. February 24, 2022. https://krishijagran.com/agripedia/cardamom-cultivation-how-to-grow-the-queen-of-spices-a-complete-guide/.

Kuta, Sarah. 2024. "Chimpanzees May Self-Medicate With Plants, Using the Forest as a Pharmacy." Smithsonian Magazine. June 24, 2024. https://www.smithsonianmag.com/smart-news/chimpanzees-may-self-medicate-with-plants-using-the-forest-as-a-pharmacy-180984593/.

Lawler, Moira. 2023. "Gotu Kola Supplement 101: Potential Benefits, Known Risks, and More." Everyday Health. July 25, 2023. https://www.everydayhealth.com/diet-nutrition/gotu-kola/guide/.

Lee, Kihyun, Sebastien Raguideau, Kimmo Sirén, Francesco Asnicar, Fabio Cumbo, Falk Hildebrand, Nicola Segata, Chang-Jun Cha, Christopher Quince. 2023. "Population-level Impacts of Antibiotic Usage on the Human Gut Microbiome." Nature Communications 14. https://doi.org/10.1038/s41467-023-36633-7.

Leech, Joe. 2023. "11 Proven Health Benefits of Ginger." Healthline. May 16, 2023. https://www.healthline.com/nutrition/11-proven-benefits-of-ginger#adding-ginger-to-the-diet.

Leichsenring, Falk, Christiane Steinert, Sven Rabung, John P. A. Ioannidis. 2023. "The Efficacy of Psychotherapies and Pharmacotherapies for Mental Disorders in Adults: An Umbrella Review and Meta-analytic Evaluation of Recent Meta-analyses. World Psychiatry 21 (1): 133-145. doi: 10.1002/wps.20941.

Leverette, Mary Marlowe. 2024. "How to Make DIY Laundry Detergent (Plus 8 Homemade Laundry Products)." The Spruce. June 10, 2024. https://www.thespruce.com/diy-laundry-products-2145722.

Levy, Jillian. 2024. "Jasmine Tea Benefits for Skin, Brain & Heart Health." Dr. Axe. May 30, 2024. https://draxe.com/nutrition/jasmine-tea-benefits/.

Levy, Jillian. 2021. "Marshmallow Root: The Ultimate Gut and Lung Protector," *Dr. Axe*, March 4, 2021. https://draxe.com/nutrition/marshmallow-root/.

Link, Rachael. 2023. "Chia Seeds Benefits: The Omega-3, Protein-Packed Superfood." Dr. Axe. October 6, 2023 https://draxe.com/nutrition/chia-seeds-benefits-side-effects/.

Link, Rachael. 2024. "Milk Thistle Benefits for the Liver, Gut & More." Dr. Axe. March 7, 2024. https://draxe.com/nutrition/milk-thistle-benefits/.

Ly, Lindy. 2011. "Make the Best Seed Starting Mix for Dirt Cheap (It"s Organic Too)." Garden Betty. March 15, 2011, https://gardenbetty.com/how-to-make-your-own-seed-starting-and-potting-mix/.

Mahr, Susan. n.d. "Cycads," Wisconsin Horticulture. https://hort.extension.wisc.edu/articles/cycads/.

Mansouri, Samaneh, Iraj Kazemi, Ahmad Reza Baghestani, Farid Zayeri, Zahra Ghorbanifar. 2020. "Evaluating the Effect of Coriandrum Sativum Syrup on Being Migraine-Free Using Mixture Models." Medical Journal of the Islamic Republic Iran 34. https://www.ncbi.nlm.nih.gov/pmc/articles/PMC7456435/

Manvitha, Karkala and Bhushan Bidya. 2014. "Aloe Vera: A Wonder Plant Its History, Cultivation and Medicinal Uses." Journal of Pharmacognosy and Phytochemistry 2 (5): 85-88 https://www.phytojournal.com/archives/2014/vol2issue5/PartB/19.1.pdf

Martinez, Apryl. 2023. "Journey into the Mystical World of Mugwort: A Guide to Harnessing its Potent Feminine Energy." Plum Brilliance. March 28, 2023. https://plumbrilliance.com/blogs/musings/journey-into-the-mystical-world-of-mugwort-a-guide-to-harnessing-its-potent-feminine-energy.

Mateo-Martín, Jimena, Guillermo Benítez, Airy Gras, Maria Molina, Victoria Reyes-García, Javier Tardío, Alonso Verde, Manuel Pardo-de-Santayana. 2023. "Cultural Importance, Availability and Conservation Status of Spanish Wild Medicinal Plants: Implications for Sustainability." People and Nature 5 (5): 1512-1525. https://doi.org/10.1002/pan3.10511.

Mayo Clinic Staff. 2024. "Alzheimer"s Disease." Mayo Clinic. July 10, 2024. https://www.mayoclinic.org/diseases-conditions/alzheimers-disease/symptoms-causes/syc-20350447.

Mayo Clinic Staff. 2023. "St. John"s Wort." Mayo Clinic. August 10, 2023. https://www.mayoclinic.org/drugs-supplements-st-johns-wort/art-20362212.

McFarland, Usha Lee. 2021. "Acknowledging its 'White Patriarchy' and Racist Past, the AMA Pledges to Dismantle Causes of Health Inequities." Stat. May 11, 2021. https://www.statnews.com/2021/05/11/ama-acknowledging-white-patriarchy-and-racist-past-pledges-to-dismantle-causes-of-health-inequities/.

Metcalf, Eric. 2023. "Stinging Nettle." WebMD. February 25, 2023. https://www.webmd.com/vitamins-and-supplements/stinging-nettle-uses-and-risks.

Moncivaiz, Aaron. 2018. "Boswellia." Healthline. October 6, 2018. https://www.healthline.com/health/boswellia.

Monjotin Nicolas, Marie Josephe Amiot, Jacques Fleurentin, Jean Michel Morel, Sylvie Raynal. 2022. "Clinical Evidence of the Benefits of

Phytonutrients in Human Health Care." Nutrients 20 (14):1712. doi: 10.3390/nu14091712.

Morrison, Oliver. 2023. "Food and Beverage Companies 'Failing to Protect Workers from Forced Labor Risks.'" Food Navigator. July 20, 2023. https://www.foodnavigator.com/Article/2023/07/20/food-and-beverage-companies-failing-to-protect-workers-from-forced-labour-risks-report.

MSKCC. 2023. "Reishi Mushroom: Purported Benefits, Side Effects & More," February 14, 2023. Memorial Sloan Kettering Cancer Center. https://www.mskcc.org/cancer-care/integrative-medicine/herbs/reishi-mushroom.

Muhammad Naoshad, Darksha Usmani, Mohammad Tarique, Huma Naz, Mohammad Ashraf, Ramesh Raliya, Shams Tabrez, Torki A. Zughaibi, Ahdab Alsaieedi, Israa J. Hakeem, Mohd Suhail. 2o22. "The Role of Natural Products and Their Multitargeted Approach to Treat Solid Cancer." Cells 11 (14): 2209. 10.3390/cells11142209.

NIH. 2023. "Ashwagandha: Is it helpful for stress, anxiety, or sleep?" National Institutes of Health, US Department of Health and Human Services. October 24, 2023. https://ods.od.nih.gov/factsheets/Ashwagandha-HealthProfessional/.

NIH. 2018. "NIH Launches HerbList, a Mobile App on Herbal Products." National Institutes of Health. June 12, 2018. https://www.nih.gov/news-events/news-releases/nih-launches-herblist-mobile-app-herbal-products.

NCHFP. 2024. "Freezing." The National Center for Home Food Preparation, University of Georgia. https://nchfp.uga.edu/how/freeze.

NCHFP. n.d. "Packaging and Storing Dried Foods," The National Center for Home Food Preparation, University of Georgia. https://nchfp.uga.edu/how/dry/drying-general/packaging-and-storing-dried-foods/.

Newman, David J. and Gordon M. Cragg. 2020. "Natural Products as Sources of Drugs of the Nearly Four Decades from 01/81 to 09/2019." Journal of Natural Products 83 (3): 770-803. https://doi.org/10.1021/acs.jnatprod.9b01285.

Nunez, Kirsten. 2023. "Keep Your Aloe Vera Gel Fresh For Longer: 5 Storage Tips + When To Toss It." MindBodyGreen. April 17, 2023. https://www.mindbodygreen.com/articles/keep-your-aloe-vera-gel-fresh-for-longer-storage-tips.

O'Leary, Michael R. 2011. "Herbal Remedies: Effects on Laboratory Tests." Laboratory Alliance 8 (39). https://www.laboratoryalliance.com/assets/Uploads/LabLines/LabLines-2010/LabLines-Winter-2010-11.pdf

OTA. n.d. "Environmental Benefits of Organic, Organic Trade Association." Organic Trade Association. https://ota.com/resources/environmental-benefits-organic

Palhares Rafael Melo, Marcela Gonçalves Drummond, Bruno Dos Santos Alves Figueiredo Brasil, Gustavo Pereira Cosenza, Maria das Graças Lins Brandão, Guilherme Oliveira. 2015. "Medicinal Plants Recommended by the World Health Organization: DNA Barcode Identification Associated with Chemical Analyses Guarantees their Quality." PLoS One 10 (5): e0127866. doi: 10.1371/journal.pone.0127866.

Pázmándi Kitti., Attila Gabor Szöllősi, Tunde Fekete. 2024. "The 'Root' Causes Hehind the Anti-inflammatory Actions of Ginger Compounds in Immune Cells." Frontiers in Immunology 15. doi: 10.3389/fimmu.2024.1400956. PMID: 39007134; PMCID: PMC11239339.

Pease Alison M, Harlan M. Krumholz, Nicholas S. Downing, Jenerius A. Aminawung, Nilay D. Shah, Joseph S. Ross. 2017. "Postapproval Studies of Drugs Initially Approved by the FDA on the Basis of Limited Evidence: Systematic Review." British Medical Journal 357: j1680. doi: 10.1136/bmj.j1680.

Perry, Megan. 2018. "The Hidden Cost of UK Food: Soil Degradation." Sustainable Food Trust. March 17, 2018. https://sustainablefoodtrust.org/news-views/the-hidden-cost-of-uk-food-soil-degradation/.

Peterson, Christine Tara, Vandana Sharma, Sasha Uchitel, Kate Denniston, Deepak Chopra, Paul J. Mills, Scott N. Peterson. 2018. "Prebiotic Potential of Herbal Medicines Used in Digestive Health and Disease."

Journal of Alternative Complementary Medicine 24 (7): 656-665. doi: 10.1089/acm.2017.0422.

Petre, Alina. 2023. "What Is Saw Palmetto? Prostate Health and Other Uses." Healthline. March 16, 2023. https://www.healthline.com/nutrition/saw-palmetto.

Petrovska, Bilijana Bauer. 2012. "Historical Review of Medicinal Plants' Usage," Pharmacognitive Review 6, (11): 1-5. doi: 10.4103/0973-7847.95849.

Philpott, Hamish, Nandurkar S., Lubel J., Gibson P.R. 2013. "Drug-induced Gastrointestinal Disorders." Frontline Gastroenterology 5 (1): 49-57. doi: 10.1136/flgastro-2013-100316.

Pietrangelo, Ann. 2024. "Which Natural Antibiotics Are the Most Effective?" Verywellhealth. January 16, 2024. https://www.verywellhealth.com/natural-antibiotics-8414343.

Potter, Rebecca. 2015. "Yarrow- Rich in Legend and Medicinal Use." Natural Ingredient.org. August 23, 2015. https://naturalingredient.org/?p=1820.

Powers, Daniel. 2022. "The 7 Best Herbs for Lung and Respiratory Health." The Botanical Institute. January 28, 2022. https://botanicalinstitute.org/herbs-for-lung-health/.

Price, Annie. 2023. "What Is Saffron? Top 6 Reasons to Add This Ancient Spice to Your Diet." Dr. Axe. March 28, 2023. https://draxe.com/nutrition/saffron/.

Price, Annie. 2024. "Burdock Root Detoxes Blood, Lymph System and Skin." Dr. Axe. June 18, 2024. https://draxe.com/nutrition/burdock-root/.

Redvers, Nicole and Be'sha Blondin. 2020. "Traditional Indigenous Medicine in North America: A Scoping Review." PLoS One 15 (8): e0237531. doi: 10.1371/journal.pone.0237531.

Reynandez, Rebecca. n.d. "How to Increase Biodiversity in Green Spaces Near You." Project Learning Tree. https://www.plt.org/educator-tips/how-increase-biodiversity.

Richter, Amy. 2024. "12 Health Benefits and Uses of Sage." Healthline. April 9, 2024. https://www.healthline.com/nutrition/sage.

Risenmay, Stacy. n.d. "Growing Herbs: Annual VS Perennial Herbs."
    https://www.notjustahousewife.net/growing-herbs-annual-vs-
    perennial-herbs/.

Ritchie, Hannah. 2022. "How Many Species Are There?"
    OurWorldInData.org/ November 30, 2022.
    https://ourworldindata.org/how-many-species-are-there.

Robinson, Molly Meri, and Xiaorui Zhang. 2011. "Traditional Medicines:
    Global Situation, Issues and Challenges." World Health Organization.
    https://www.utep.edu/herbal-safety/herbal-
    facts/files/wms_ch18_wtraditionalmed-2011.pdf

Semeco, Arlene. 2023. "7 Proven Benefits of Ginseng." Healthline. December
    15, 2023. https://www.healthline.com/nutrition/ginseng-benefits

Sharma, Tarang, Louise Schow Guski, Nana Freund, Peter C. Gøtzsche. 2016.
    "Suicidality and Aggression During Antidepressant Treatment:
    Systematic Review and Meta-analyses Based on Clinical Study
    Reports." British Medical Journal 352. doi: 10.1136/bmj.i65.

Siwek, Marcin., Jaroslaw Woroń, Anna Wrzosek, Jaroslaw Gupało, Adrian
    Andrzej Chrobak. 2023. "Harder, Better, Faster, Stronger?
    Retrospective Chart Review of Adverse Events of Interactions
    Between Adaptogens and Antidepressant Drugs." Frontiers in
    Pharmacology 14. doi: 10.3389/fphar.2023.1271776.

Stallard, Esme. 2023. "What is Biodiversity and How Are We Protecting It?"
    BBC News. April 21, 2023. https://www.bbc.com/news/explainers-
    60823267.

Stankiewicz, Karen. 2022. "Herbs to Plant Together: Companion Planting
    with Herbs." Utopia. March 11, 2022.
    https://utopia.org/guide/herbs-to-plant-together-companion-
    planting-with-herbs/.

Svedi, Robin. 2021. "Herb Garden Guide: Everything You Need To Know
    About Growing Herbs." Gardening Know How. June 15, 2021.
    https://www.gardeningknowhow.com/edible/herbs/hgen/general-
    care-for-your-herb-garden.htm.

Sweet, Hannah. n.d. "How to Forage: All You Need to Know." Eat The Planet.
    https://eattheplanet.org/how-to-forage-all-you-need-to-know/.

Talerico, Deanna. 2022. "How to Make Medicinal Herb Infused Oil: Two Ways." HomesteadandChill.com. November 2, 2022. https://homesteadandchill.com/medicinal-herb-infused-oil-tutorial/.

Talkspace. 2023. "Valerian Root For Anxiety: Does it Work?" Talkspace. September 28, 2023. https://www.talkspace.com/mental-health/conditions/articles/valerian-root-for-anxiety/.

Temkin, Alexis M., Samara L. Geller, Sydney A. Swanson, Nneka S. Leiba, Olga V. Naidenko, David Q. Andrews. 2023. "Volatile Organic Compounds Emitted by Conventional and 'Green' Cleaning Products in the U.S. Market." Chemosphere 341. https://doi.org/10.1016/j.chemosphere.2023.139570.

Terry, Will. 2023. "The Spiritual Meaning Of Hawthorn: Symbolism, Rituals, And Healing Properties. "Garvillo. October 9, 2023. https://garvillo.com/hawthorn-spiritual-meaning/.

Thomas, Liji. 2021. "Plant-Based Drugs and Medicine." News Medical Life Sciences. December 23, 2021. https://www.news-medical.net/health/Plant-Based-Drugs-and-Medicines.aspx#:~:.

Thumann, Timo A., Eva-Maria Pferschy-Wenzig, Chistine Moissl-Eichinger, Rudolf Bauer. 2019. "The Role of Gut Microbiota for the Activity of Medicinal Plants Traditionally Used in the European Union for Gastrointestinal Disorders." Journal of Ethnopharmacology 245: 112153. doi: 10.1016/j.jep.2019.112153.

Timmins Malek, Amy. 2019. "The Medicinal Uses and Health Benefits of Red Clover." Wishgarden Herbs. September 26, 2019. https://www.wishgardenherbs.com/blogs/wishgarden/red-clover.

Timmons, Greg. 2023. "Hippocrates." Biography.com. August 9, 2023. https://www.biography.com/scholars-educators/hippocrates.

Timmons, Jessica. 2020. "The Pitta Dosha: How To Eat, Exercise & De-Stress To Keep It In Check." Mind Body Green Health. September 28, 2020. https://www.mindbodygreen.com/articles/pitta-dosha-understanding-this-ayurveda-type-tips.

Tóth-Mészáros, Andrea, Gantsetseg Garmaa, Peter Hegyi, Andras Bánvölgyi, Bank Fenyves, Peter Fehérvári, Andrea Harnos, Dorottya Gergő, Uyen Nguyen Do To, Dezső Csupor. 2023. "The Effect of Adaptogenic

Plants on Stress: A Systematic Review and Meta-Analysis." Journal of Functional Foods 108. https://doi.org/10.1016/j.jff.2023.105695.

Touwaide, Alain and Emanuela Appetiti. 2023. "Herbs in History: Valerian." American Herbal Products Association, July 2023. https://www.ahpa.org/herbs_in_history_valerian.

UCLA Health, 2023. "What are Phytochemicals (and Why Should You Eat More of Them)." UCLA Health. May 10, 2023. https://www.uclahealth.org/news/article/what-are-phytochemicals-and-why-should-you-eat-more-them.

UNEP. 2021. "Our Global Food System is the Primary Driver of Biodiversity Loss." United Nations Environment Programme. February 3, 2021. https://www.unep.org/news-and-stories/press-release/our-global-food-system-primary-driver-biodiversity-loss.

Upham, Becky. 2023. "Conventional Cleaning Products Emit Hundreds of Hazardous Chemicals." Everyday Health. September 13, 2023. https://www.everydayhealth.com/healthy-home/conventional-cleaning-products-emit-hundreds-of-hazardous-chemicals/.

USDA. n.d. "About the Organics Standards," United States Department of Agriculture. https://www.ams.usda.gov/grades-standards/organic-standards.

USDA. n.d. "Understanding Food Quality Labels." United States Department of Agriculture. https://www.ams.usda.gov/sites/default/files/media/AMSProductLabelFactsheet.pdf.

Veeresham Ciddi. 2012. "Natural Products Derived from Plants as a Source of Drugs." Journal of Advanced Pharmaceutical Technology and Research 3 (4):200-1. doi: 10.4103/2231-4040.104709.

Vialli, Kyle. 2024. "The Shocking Truth About Aloe Vera (And How to Remove the Latex)." Kylevialli.com. https://www.kylevialli.com/blog/the-truth-about-aloe-vera.

Wahbeh, Helane, Angela Senders, Rachel Neuendorf, Julien Cayton. 2014. "Complementary and Alternative Medicine for Posttraumatic Stress Disorder Symptoms: A Systematic Review." Journal of Evidence Based

Complementary Alternative Medicine 19 (3): 161-175. doi:
10.1177/2156587214525403.

Wang, Guanqiang, Tongren Ding, Lianzhong Ai. 2024. "Editorial: Effects and
Mechanisms of Probiotics, Prebiotics, Synbiotics and Postbiotics on
Intestinal Health and Disease." Frontiers in Cellular and Infection
Microbiology 14: 1430312. doi: 10.3389/fcimb.2024.1430312.

WebMD Editorial Contributors. 2023. "Health Benefits of Black Elderberry."
WebMD. March 23, 2023. https://www.webmd.com/diet/health-
benefits-black-elderberry.

WEF. 2021. "The Global Eco-Wakening: How Consumers are Driving
Sustainability." World Economic Forum. May 18, 2021.
https://www.weforum.org/agenda/2021/05/eco-wakening-
consumers-driving-sustainability/.

Willson, Mark. 2024. "Anti-Anxiety Medication Use Soars in Past Decade."
Anxiety.org. March 3, 2024. https://www.anxiety.org/antianxiety-
medication-use-soars-in-past-decade.

World Health Organization. 2013. "WHO Traditional Medicine Strategy:
2014-2023." World Health Organization. May 15, 2013.
https://www.who.int/publications/i/item/9789241506096.

World Health Organization. 2023. "The First WHO Traditional Medicine
Global Summit." August 17, 2023.

Printed in Great Britain
by Amazon

58323978R00089